T0239143

"As a seasoned academic emergency physician with decades of ambulance and wilderness prehospital experience, I have seen the critical role that hypnosis can play in these settings. In their groundbreaking book, the authors draw on their extensive background in both the EMS and psychology to provide a comprehensive guide to using hypnotic communication techniques in prehospital care. Incorporating the latest research in hypnosis, they provide practical, real-world strategies, practical tips, and expert advice. This book is an essential resource for EMS responders."

Kenneth V. Iserson, *M.D., MBA, FACEP, FAAEM, FIFEM, Professor Emeritus, Department of Emergency Medicine, University of Arizona College of Medicine*

"This material presents both an opportunity and a challenge to all prehospital care personnel. The opportunity is to develop patient communication at a level previously unknown, a level that may enhance positive and possibly lifesaving physiological responses. The challenge is to break through the barriers of bias, preconception, and mindset that deter objective evaluation."

Thomas Elmendorf, *M.D., Past President of the California Medical Association*

"*Hypnotic Communication in Emergency Medical Settings* is an essential resource for medical professionals seeking to improve patient outcomes. The authors provide practical techniques for using hypnotic communication to calm patients and reduce anxiety during emergency situations. This book is a valuable addition to any medical library and a must-read for those working in emergency medicine. Highly recommended!"

Joseph Varon, *MD, FACP, FCCP, FCCM, FRSM, Clinical Professor, University of Houston College of Medicine; Associate Dean, Caribbean Medical University; Editor-in-Chief for the journals 'Critical Care and Shock' and 'Current Respiratory Medicine Reviews'.*

Hypnotic Communication in Emergency Medical Settings

This fascinating book demonstrates how hypnotic communication has the potential to improve patient outcomes in emergency care, integrating insights on the connection between mind and body for paramedics and other first responders.

Providing a step-by-step guide to using these skills around a range of contexts, from managing pain to cardiovascular emergencies to burns to respiratory distress, the book asks paramedics and first responders to become aware of what they say to patients, as well as how they say it. It offers ways to allow targeted communication to complement standard medical procedures, creating a symbiotic rapport that will provide the basis for an improved outcome for the patient.

Fully referenced and based on a robust range of evidence, the book is written by an active paramedic with over 20 years' experience with a Ph.D. in Human Development with a focus on paramedic decision-making; and a professor with doctorates in Health Psychology and Education who field tested the skills as a professional EMT. This book will interest any professional working in emergency care, including paramedics, EMTs, trauma nurses, and psychiatric nurses.

Four Arrows (Don Trent Jacobs), Ph.D., Ed.D., is the author of more than 20 books on wellness, education, and Indigenous worldview. A former firefighter/EMT and Vice President of the Northern California Society of Clinical Hypnosis, he is currently a professor of educational leadership for change at Fielding Graduate University. Reach him at www.fourarrowsbooks.com.

Bram Duffee, Ph.D., is a full-time paramedic, researcher, and speaker from Houston, Texas, who teaches interpersonal communication and leadership. As a specialist in conversation analysis, he examines paramedic interactions with the goal of improving emergency healthcare. He is currently a Research Fellow with the Institute for Social Innovation at Fielding Graduate University. Reach him at www.BramDuffee.com.

Hypnotic Communication in Emergency Medical Settings

For Life-Saving and Therapeutic Outcomes

**Four Arrows (Don Trent Jacobs)
and Bram Duffee**

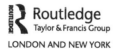

LONDON AND NEW YORK

Designed cover image: © Getty Images

First published 2024
by Routledge
4 Park Square, Milton Park, Abingdon, Oxon OX14 4RN

and by Routledge
605 Third Avenue, New York, NY 10158

Routledge is an imprint of the Taylor & Francis Group, an informa business

British Library Cataloguing-in-Publication Data
A catalogue record for this book is available from the British Library

ISBN: 978-1-032-55349-8 (hbk)
ISBN: 978-1-032-36002-7 (pbk)
ISBN: 978-1-003-43026-1 (ebk)

DOI: 10.4324/9781003430261

Typeset in Times New Roman
by codeMantra

Contents

Preface

A non-fiction book's preface usually tells why authors are motivated to write about their topic. At the end of this section, we (Bram and Four Arrows) communicate our personal reasons for writing this book. For now, we begin with our shared belief that words spoken to an emergency medical or trauma victim within the first hour or so have the potential to make a difference that will save lives, alleviate suffering, and initiate healing. We have learned this mostly from our nearly 40 years of combined field experience in emergency medicine and hypnosis. However, as academics, both of us with research doctorates, we also know the research that supports this belief. Although we minimize academic jargon supportive citations in the rest of the book, we offer some studies here that refer to such research. The following abstracts are examples of many that prove how hypnosis can be an effective medical intervention for the kinds of medical emergencies that occur worldwide, many of which we address in this text.

First, we offer our working definition of hypnosis so you know what these research conclusions really show. The word "hypnosis" can refer to an altered consciousness that makes a person able to activate responses differently from normal consciousness. More specifically, during this alternative consciousness, there are cognitive/sensory changes in the frequency of the brain as well as nervous system oscillations. Lower frequencies, such as theta oscillations, seem to facilitate responding to mental or verbal directives or suggestions, and at the same time, an effect on a higher frequency (gamma) links different circuits in the brain to create physiological responses such as a reduction in pain sensation.[i] Researchers from the University of Turku, Finland, also found that during hypnosis the brain shifted to a state where individual brain regions acted more independently of each other.[ii] It is interesting to note that for decades, scientists refused to believe that hypnosis actually changed brain activity. However, with improved technologies, they have proven that the ability of hypnosis to control pain and reduce anxiety is clearly associated with functional changes in brain activity. For example, a systematic review of 10, 404 peer-reviewed articles identified significant differences in brain activity during hypnosis relating to location and frequency.[iii]

The word "hypnosis" is also used to describe the process by which such neurological changes take place, whether in hetero-hypnosis or self-hypnosis. Here, scientific research offers little beyond describing the particular techniques used in various experiments because there are so many approaches. There are common threads in clinical hypnosis and in stage hypnosis we could describe. However, our goal in this book is not to teach hypnotic induction techniques per se. It is to convince readers that spontaneous states of hypnotic consciousness occur during trauma that makes whatever is said to a patient by a first responder a potential hypnotic suggestion. After presenting the following list of abstracts that support this assertion, we have more to say about spontaneous hypnosis and why our belief in it has motivated us to write this text.

Abstract #1: Hypnosis in Emergency Medicine: Let's Change Our Habits!

The effectiveness of hypnosis in the management of pain and anxiety has been widely demonstrated today. While this technique is commonly used in anesthesia and psychiatry, its use in emergencies is still poorly developed. The fields of application in hospital and extra-hospital emergency are however multiple, and, contrary to popular belief, emergencies are the ideal place for the practice of hypnosis. Hypnosis is a reliable, safe, effective, and inexpensive technique that any caregiver can learn. It strengthens the caregiver-patient relationship and helps us to treat differently, more humanly, and more serenely.[iv]

Abstract #2: The Use of Hypnosis in Emergency Medicine

Hypnosis can be a useful adjunct in the emergency department setting. Its efficacy in various clinical applications has been replicated in controlled studies. Application to burns, pain, pediatric procedures, surgery, psychiatric presentations (e.g., coma, somatoform disorder, anxiety, and posttraumatic stress), and obstetric situations (e.g., hyperemesis, labor, and delivery) are described.[v]

Abstract #3: Hypnosis as Emergency Treatment for the Mentally Ill and in Disaster Situations

For an individual as well as for a group of people, a disaster may be associated with acute physical and/or mental collapse. As well as taking swift physical measures in such situations, it may be necessary to give equally rapid mental help. To this end, hypnosis, or more properly, hetero-hypnosis is an important method.[vi]

Abstract #4: Adjunctive Non-pharmacological Analgesia for Invasive Medical Procedures

A Randomized Trial

Non-pharmacological behavioral adjuncts have been suggested as efficient safe means in reducing discomfort and adverse effects during medical procedures. Non-pharmacological adjuncts have a positive effect on patients' comfort levels compared with standard conditions despite the use of half the analgesic and anti-anxiety medication. The trend toward less pain and anxiety over time, found with structured attention, reached significance with the addition of hypnosis.[vii]

Abstract #5: Autonomic Cardiac Reactivity to Painful Procedures

Under Hypnosis in Pediatric Emergencies

The aim of this study was to investigate the impact of hypnosis on pain perception in children during clinical procedures. Specifically, the researchers examined the autonomic responses of pediatric patients undergoing sutures under hypnosis in emergency settings. Pain sensation is characterized by abrupt changes in central nervous system activity producing autonomic reactivity. Time-frequency analysis was applied on RR intervals (heart rate intervals, or RRI) to estimate parasympathetic reactivity. To conclude, hypnosis in pediatric emergencies reduces sympathetic cardiac pain reactivity and could be a marker of pain relief under hypnosis, while parasympathetic activity seems to be a better marker of hypnosis.[viii]

Abstract #6: Hypnosis for Asthma: A Controlled Trial

An investigation of hypnosis in asthma was made among patients aged 10 to 60 years with paroxysmal attacks of wheezing or tight chest capable of relief by bronchodilators. Independent clinical assessors considered asthma to be "much better" in 59% of the hypnosis group and in 43% of the control group, the difference being significant. There was little difference between the sexes. Physicians with previous experience of hypnosis obtained significantly better results than did those without such experience.[ix]

Abstract #7: The Hypnotic Control of Blood Flow and Pain

Case histories show that hypnosis can control massive bleeding and pain, and it can remove warts, probably by stopping blood flow to them. We propose that blood flow to cancerous tumors can likewise be controlled, which could destroy them outright, or which control could be a useful adjunct to chemo- or radiotherapy.[x]

Abstract #8: Use of Relaxation and Hypnosis in Lowering High Blood Pressure

Investigation was made to determine whether high blood pressure (hypertension) could be lowered through (a) muscular relaxation and (b) hypnosis. Six non-medicated hypertensive patients were used as controls, while another six served as treatment group receiving muscular relaxation and hypnosis procedures. Nine patients on stabilized anti-hypertensive medication also received muscular relaxation and hypnosis procedures. Significant lowering of both systolic and diastolic pressures was obtained in both the no-drug and drug groups receiving treatment, but there was no significant reduction in the control group. Hypertensive levels were reduced through muscular relaxation and completely eliminated during hypnosis. Instruction was given in self-relaxation and self-hypnosis to promote the continuation of beneficial effects beyond hospitalization.[xi]

Abstract #9: An Hypnotic Suggestion: Review of Hypnosis for Clinical Emergency Care

Hypnosis has been used in medicine for nearly 250 years. Yet, emergency clinicians rarely use it in emergency departments or prehospital settings. This review describes hypnosis, its historical use in medicine, several neurophysiologic studies of the procedure, its uses, and potential uses in emergency care. It suggests methods of increasing its use in emergency care. Although it is safe, fast, and cost-effective, emergency clinicians rarely use hypnosis. This is due, in part, to the myths surrounding hypnosis and its association with alternative-complementary medicine. Genuine barriers to its increased clinical use include a lack of assured effectiveness and a lack of training and training requirements. Based on the results of further research, hypnosis could become a powerful and safe nonpharmacologic addition to the emergency clinician's armamentarium, with the potential to enhance patient care in emergency medicine, prehospital care, and remote medical settings.[xii]

In this last abstract, the author notes the unfortunate fact that the use of hypnosis for medical emergencies is rarely used—owing to myths about it and a lack of training in it. We intend for this book to address both of these restraints to saving lives. We know that with the kind of practical "training" we offer, more and more first responders and EMS agencies will want to start bringing our communication strategies that recognize spontaneous hypnosis in victims. Two studies reveal that learning about this power of words does motivate professional medics. Perhaps it is because they intuitively realize that they have always had this power, though no one had named it for them. One study shows how nurses changed their communication behaviors after learning about hypnotic techniques designed to manage pain in children undergoing medical procedures.[xiii]

Another is a soon-to-be-published doctoral dissertation by Michael Moates. He surveyed over a thousand professional first responders about whether they thought their words could potentially have a positive hypnotic effect on treatment outcomes. Then, he had them read a short description of the phenomenon. Over 50% changed from a negative response to a positive one.

Thomas Elmendorf, M.D., former past president of the California Medical Association, refers to the barriers to bringing this book's message to the fore of emergency medicine. Written in 1991 for the original manuscript that inspired this publication, he writes:

> The material presents both an opportunity and a challenge to all prehospital care personnel. The opportunity is to develop patient communication at a level previously unknown, a level that may enhance positive and possibly lifesaving physiological responses. The challenge is to break through the barriers of bias, preconception, and mind-set that deter objective evaluation.

Spontaneous Hypnosis

Another important thing to note in the abstracts cited above is that they all involved hypnotic induction techniques. Whether or not that was necessary for those related to medical emergencies is not discussed. This brings us back to the idea of spontaneous hypnosis. Our book's approach assumes that the emergency victim is spontaneously in a state of hypnosis and that no "induction" per se is necessary. The American Academy of Orthopedic Surgeons apparently agrees with this assumption when in their 4th edition of Care and Transportation of the Sick and Injured, the author says that first responders must be "extremely careful about what is said at the scene. During periods of great stress, words that seem immaterial or are uttered in jest might become fixed in the patient's mind and cause untold harm. Conversation at the scene must be appropriate." Of course, they do not explain why, and in this and all of their many subsequent editions, they go no further than to tell their readers that a first step in care management is to "calm and reassure" the patient.

Not giving attention in academic studies to spontaneous hypnosis is understandable. If intentionality in a laboratory or hospital for hypnosis existed, it could not be spontaneous. This said, there is sufficient anecdotal evidence for the existence and importance of spontaneous hypnosis for us to feel this book can save many lives and alleviate much suffering. Arreed F. Barabasz is someone who agrees with us. Before we cite his position on this, we note his exceptional credentials. At only 23 years of age, Arreed Franz Barabasz, EdD, Ph.D., American Board of Professional Psychology (ABPP), completed his first doctoral degree in Counseling Psychology at State University of New York at Albany. His Ph.D. in Clinical and Human Experimental Psychology is from the University of Canterbury, New Zealand, where he conducted the first studies of EEG and Hypnosis in Antarctica. His postdoctoral Clinical Fellowship was at Harvard Medical School & Massachusetts General Hospital. Dr. Barbasz is a Full Professor and Director of the Laboratory of Hypnosis Research at Washington State University. He was an Associate Professor of Psychology at Harvard University Medical School prior to his current position. Dr. Barabasz is the Editor of the *International Journal of Clinical and Experimental Hypnosis (IJCEH)* (2002–2018), the highest citation index-ranked journal in the field. He is a licensed psychologist and Diplomat of the ABPP—the highest distinction in professional psychology. Arreed holds a Fellow status for "Outstanding and unusual contributions to the science and practice of psychology," from the American Psychological Association (APA).

Barbasz's work is important to mention in our preface if only to show we are not the only ones concerned about the lack of attention given to the phenomenon of spontaneous hypnosis. In an article criticizing the APA for omitting spontaneous hypnosis in its newest definition of hypnosis,[xiv] he says that "A definition that fails to include spontaneous hypnosis gives researchers 'license' to fail to experimentally control for the potential influence of this variable on their findings." He gives an example where in one study that has been influencing hypnotic research for decades failed to discuss one of five subjects in spontaneous hypnosis that had the same hypnotic responses as those who were professionally hypnotized. He continues explaining how hypnosis literature is littered with studies that ignore potential occurrences of spontaneous hypnosis. "It is naïve for a clinician to assume that if he or she is not formally using hypnosis it does not occur." He also says that "Exposure to a traumatic event is a common excitation leading to spontaneous hypnosis."

Another article referring to spontaneous hypnosis comes from psychiatry law and forensics. The author, John O. Beahrs, M.D. says "Hypnotic-like phenomena and transactions occur spontaneously, in either covert or overt forms." He describes four overlapping types of spontaneous hypnosis. In one section titled "Trauma and Spontaneous Hypnosis," he says "the experience of a catastrophic stressor is nearly always accompanied by profound alternations in subjective volition, sense of time, and other cognitive/perceptual alterations that meet criteria for overt hypnotic states."[xv]

Our Individual Personal Reasons for Writing This Book

Don Trent Jacobs, Ph.D., Ed.D., aka Wahinkpe Topa (Four Arrows)
I learned about the potential benefits of hypnotic language at the emergency scene long ago in the 1980s. Simultaneously renewing my EMT training; taking a course in hypnotherapy during my doctoral work in health psychology; responding to many medical emergencies as a firefighter/EMT for the Marin County Fire Department; and training wild mustangs (Search YouTube for "Wild Horse Hypnotist), I started using "emergency hypnosis" on some calls. While working as an

EMT, I got my doctorate in health psychology. Eventually, I quit the fire service and started a hypnotherapy practice. I became the vice president of the Northern California Society of Clinical Hypnosis and taught hypnosis at UC Berkeley as an adjunct for Marriage, Family and Child Counseling hypnosis certification.

During the transition from EMT to clinical hypnotherapist, I created a video[1] with a number of respected physicians and my team of EMTs who were using it. I think that it might be the first introduction of this topic to the world. Norman Cousins, author of Anatomy of an Illness, saw the video. At the time, he was doing research at UCLA with actors and actresses "imagining" different emotions to see how they influenced their biochemistry. He contacted me and suggested to write a book about it. I created the manuscript and sent it out for endorsements. I received the following for the original manuscript:

"This book should be in every person's library and should be studied carefully by all of us...the knowledge we absorb here may save many lives."
David Cheek, M.D., author of The Psychobiology
of Mind/Body Healing

"This book presents field tested techniques proven to have an invaluable influence on patient recovery."
Journal of Emergency Services

"This approach presents an opportunity to develop patient care at a level previously unknown."
Thomas Elmendorf, M.D. (former) president of the
California Medical Association

"This material is on the cutting edge of an exciting an innovative approach to pre-hospital care."
Benny Cooper, Director of Emergency Medical
Training at Murray State University

"...It provides valuable information on multiple aspects of the patient/physician relationship. I cannot imagine any patient or emergency care provider who would not benefit from this approach to treating a person in trauma."
Norman Cousins, UCLA School of Medicine, author
of Anatomy of an Illness

Unfortunately, the 1980s and early 1990s were the right time for my book. I say "unfortunately" because I know that many lives could have been positively affected if this book had been available to first responders over these many years. In the era we are now facing, with a likely increase in medical emergencies, perhaps the world will now embrace this life-saving, easy-to-use form of communication as an adjunct to standard first-aid and emergency medical care everywhere.

This said, there still exists much skepticism about the hypnosis phenomenon. Too many see it as something "make believe" that does not really relate to a biological transformation in nervous system functioning. Here are just three studies that can help clarify that hypnosis is real and proven clinically:

Antonio Del Casale, Stefano Ferracuti, Chiara Rapinesi, Daniele Serata, Gabriele Sani, Valeria Savoja, Georgios D. Kotzalidis, Roberto Tatarelli & Paolo Girardi. (2012). Neurocognition under hypnosis: Findings from recent functional neuroimaging studies, *International Journal of Clinical and Experimental Hypnosis,* **60(3), 286–317, DOI: 10.1080/00207144.2012.675295**

Study 1: Brain scans show that when people are hypnotized, the front part of their brain helps them to pay more attention. This part also helps to separate out different thoughts. Other parts of the brain also change and help with seeing things differently. Finally, there are changes in the back part of the brain which help with how people act on different suggestions.

Kosslyn, S. M., Thompson, W. L., Costantini-Ferrando, M. F., Alpert, N. M., & Spiegel, D. (2000). Hypnotic visual illusion alters color processing in the brain. *American Journal of Psychiatry,* **157(8), 1279–1284.**

Study 2: When people were hypnotized, the left and right sides of their brains lit up when they were asked to see color. But the same parts got less light when they were asked to see gray. This only happened during hypnosis, and it was different on the left side than on the right side. People who can be hypnotized can have changes in their feelings and thoughts that show up in their brains. This means hypnosis is real and not just pretending.

Tuominen, J., Kallio, S., Kaasinen, V., & Railo, H. (2021). Segregated brain state during hypnosis. *Neuroscience of Consciousness,* **2021(1), niab002.**

Study 3: This group conducted an experiment to investigate how the brain responds to a type of magnetic energy that affects electrical activity. The experiment revealed that when an individual is prescribed a single-word suggestion, the connections in the brain are altered, and it becomes difficult for stronger signals to be transmitted between different areas. The results of this experiment suggest that hypnosis can alter events occurring in the brain, possibly influencing how people react under hypnosis.

As an Indigenous-based scholar, I believe in the Indigenous idea that words are sacred vibrations. Traditional Indigenous cultures and all of our distant precolonial ancestors knew the power of trance-based learning and healing and used it regularly. The reader can learn more about this in other books that I have written, including Point of Departure, Primal Awareness, and Restoring our Kinship Worldview.

Bram Duffee

In 1998, I became a paramedic at 19 and was given a great deal of responsibility at a young age. I was very young to be doing a job that requires strong leadership, and I found out quickly that my words and how I said those words influence everyone in the environment. This is especially true on the scene of an emergency when everyone is already experiencing some degree of stress. So, when I am communicating to my crew on the scene or to the dispatcher by radio, they are listening for how to interpret the situation based on nonverbal parts of my message like tone and volume. If I am stressed or emotional or fearful, they might know, and I did not want to ever seem as if I could not handle the stress because of my age. Similarly, if my coworkers or the bystanders could tell that the person in charge is stressed, then of course that stress transfers to the patient as well. To mitigate that issue early on, I focused on adhering to the principles that I was taught as an Eagle Scout that influenced my professional look, trim haircut, and always perfect uniform.

I realized that my image makes a real difference in my ability to provide the best medical care. But, even with this realization, and giving maximum effort to be effective as a clinician, I still had patient encounters where the patient died because they refused to go to the hospital by ambulance. The most common scenario would be an older man who has severe heart attack symptoms and emphatically refuses to go to the hospital even with my medical opinion and the urging of family. I know the patient was refusing to go to the hospital because they are in denial and afraid. So, refusing to acknowledge the situation by getting treatment or going to the hospital would help the patient feel as if they were maintaining control. In some cases, I had very argumentative interactions with patients because I was able to bluntly tell them what I thought was wrong with them and how I wanted to fix it. I would be in situations where the patient might die if I am not successfully persuasive enough to convince them to go with me to the hospital. These "arguments" I was having, usually with older men in rural settings, were something I was interested in studying.

While working as a paramedic I studied conversational analysis under Phillip Glenn, Ph.D. my first master's degree in speech communication. My initial orientation to analyzing conversation was through the deep study of one particular aspect of language, laughter. I used transcription equipment that advanced a tape by foot pedal to manually type each utterance of sound I recorded. Laughter was not just "LOL." I began to understand the unlimited ways that someone could laugh, and how different each utterance can be. "Hhaa," "haa ha," "HAAAAaha," and "Haaahaa" have much different sounds, for example. Through this narrow view of understanding, a small aspect of language was born a big awareness of the world involving nonverbal communication. It helped me understand other forms of nonverbal communication and how they influence the meaning of messages.

During this time, I also taught a communications class at Southern Illinois University where I was able to better explore these concepts with my students. We were able to research the everyday environment to find examples of how voice can communicate through pitch, rate, volume, intonation, pauses, and quality. We also researched and studied the body and how to communicate different messages based on distance and orientation to the other person as well as facial expressions, posture, and touch. These insights influenced how I approached my patients as a paramedic and helped me think about how to best interact with them in stressful situations.

I was now fueled with a quest for paramedic clinical excellence, had a new orientation to interpersonal communication, and possessed a strong desire to convince my patients to make good medical decisions. This led to my master's thesis "Incongruent perceptions and training styles: The paramedic in conflict with the emotionally charged bystander" that was published and then, along with Nilanjana Bardhan, Ph.D., presented at the 2007 National Communication Association Conference in Chicago. The study showed that paramedics usually use a conflict style that is determined in the moment. This adaptability is helpful. But poor communication choices can still plague the inexperienced paramedic because conflict training for patient interactions is not part of the paramedic curriculum.

While completing the coursework for my Ph.D. in Human Development, I did a 911 call on the ambulance as a paramedic where I took care of a baby girl who was very violently tortured, molested, and stabbed with the intention of causing death. It was one of those calls where we had multiple victims, limited resources, and the worst patient needed urgent transport without delay. This baby was now actively dying and alone in the back of the ambulance with me as the only person who can take action to prevent death. This was the worst moment of my paramedic career. I knew exactly what needed to be done. I was only one person with two hands and one brain but nothing could be done good enough or fast enough. The case was so serious, and we had a police escort pushing traffic away from the front of the ambulance. I was emotional as I told my partner who was driving that he needed to literally drive as fast as possible and break all the rules necessary because speed is the only thing that can save her. My patient needed to breathe but there were too many stab wounds to the lungs that were too large to seal off while at the same time I had to keep the baby breathing. It was literally a case up to the last second before death when I did the hospital handoff. I will never forget the face of the doctor who took the baby from me and started emergency surgery right there in the emergency room. The call was over for me. The baby did not die in real life, but the pressure of the event was so overwhelming that I had flashbacks of the event when I was awake and ended up being diagnosed with PTSD.

It was during my PTSD recovery that I began to read about how the mind-body connection works to influence health. I enthusiastically read *Hypnosis without Trance* by Tripp and *The Worst Is Over* by Acosta and Prager who studied under Four Arrows. As luck would have it, Four Arrows was a professor in my Ph.D. program, and we found many similar interests and philosophies, especially about how people communicate during emergencies.

This led to a research project for my dissertation titled "High-stress high-consequence emergency medical decision making: Paramedics seeking a differential diagnosis." This study helped define and explain the high-stress, high-consequence situations encountered by paramedics. Results show that paramedics require lengthy on-the-job experience to gain the skills necessary to create mental models for making good decisions under stress. These mental models help experienced paramedics be more intuitive. This need for experience is so important that I suggest the need for development in areas like virtual reality (VR) simulation training similar to the training required for airline pilots.

Today, I still practice as a full-time paramedic where I continue to develop my own clinical communication competency. As you read this book, I invite you to join me in this life-long pursuit of communication excellence in emergency healthcare.

Note

1 The original video can be viewed on Youtube at https://youtu.be/iVIMoE9scOA

References

i   Jensen, M.P., Adachi, T., & Hakimian, S. (January, 2015). Brain oscillations, hypnosis and hypnotizability. *American Journal of Clinical Hypnosis*, 57(3). https://www.ncbi.nlm.nih.gov/pmc/articles/PMC4361031/

ii   Tuominen, J., Kallio, S., Kaasinen, V., & Railo, H. (2021). Segregated brain state during hypnosis. *Neuroscience of Consciousness*, 2021(1). https://doi.org/10.1093/nc/niab002

iii   Wolf, T.G., Faerber, K.A., Rummel, C., Haisband, U., & Camppus, G. (January, 2022). Functional changes in brain activity using hypnosis: A systematic review. *Brain Science.* https://www.ncbi.nlm.nih.gov/pmc/articles/PMC8773773/

iv   Schmutz, T., Ribordy, V., Aim, P., Pham-Dinh, C., Braun, F., & Guler, N. (September, 2020). Hypnosis in emergency medicine: let's change our habits! *Revue Medicale Suisse*, 16(707), 1757–1762. https://europepmc.org/article/med/32969613

v   Peebles-Kleiger, M.J. (May, 2000). The use of hypnosis in emergency medicine. *Emergency Medicine Clinical North America*, 18(2), 327–338. https://pubmed.ncbi.nlm.nih.gov/10767888/

vi   Langen, D. (1980). Hypnosis as emergency treatment for the mentally ill and in disaster situations. In: Frey, R., & Safar, P. (eds) *Resuscitation and Life Support in Disasters Relief of Pain and Suffering in Disaster Situations. Disaster Medicine*, vol. 2. Springer, Berlin, Heidelberg. https://doi.org/10.1007/978-3-642-67095-4_29

vii   Lang, E.V., Benotsch, E.G., Fick, L.J., Lutgendorf, S., et al. (April, 2000). Adjunctive non-pharmacological analgesia for invasive medical procedures: A randomised trial. *The Lancet*, 355(9214), 1486–1490. https://fielding-summon-serialssolutions-com.fgul.idm.oclc.org/?#!/search?ho=t&include.ft.matches=t&l=en&q=Hypnosis%20Medical%20Emergencies

viii Excoffier, J., Pichot, V., Cantais, A. et al. (January, 2020). Autonomic cardiac reactivity to painful procedures under hypnosis in pediatric emergencies. *The American Journal of Clinical Hypnosis*, 62(3), 267–281. https://doi.org/10.1080/00 029157.2018.1564013.

ix Members of the Hypnotherapy in Asthma Subcommittee (October, 1968). Hypnosis for asthma- a controlled trial. A report to the Research Committee of the British Tuberculosis Association. *British Medical Journal*, 4(5623), 71–76. https://www. ncbi.nlm.nih.gov/pmc/articles/PMC1912142/

x Clawson, A., & Swade, R. (1975). The hypnotic control of bood flow and pain. "*American Journal of Clinical Hypnosis*, 17:3, 160–169, DOI: 10.1080/00029157.1 975.10403735

xi Deabler, H.L., Fidel, E., Dillenkoffer, R.L., & Elder, S.T. (1973). The use of relaxation and hypnosis in lowering high blood pressure. *American Journal of Clinical Hypnosis*, 16(2), 75–83. https://doi.org/10.1080/00029157.1973.10403656

xii Iserson, K.V. (April, 2014). An hypnotic suggestion: Review of hypnosis for clinical emergency care. *Journal of Emergency Medicine*, 46(4), 588–596. https://pubmed. ncbi.nlm.nih.gov/24472351/

xiii Aramideh, J., Ogez, D., Mizrahi, T., Marie-Claude, C., Plante, C. et al. (August, 2020). Do professionals change their communication behaviours following a training in hypnosis-derived communication? *Complementary Therapies in Medicine*, 52. https://www.proquest.com/docview/2443480457?accountid=10868&parentSe ssionId=tRo7aRLapq3fPeJJWpJE%2BcDOJuVurAgkUBFVomWPtZY%3D&pq-o rigsite=summon

xiv Barabasz, A.F., & Barbasz, M.R. (2015). The new APA definition of hypnosis: Spontaneous hypnosis MIA. *American Journal of Clinical Hypnosis*, 57(4), 459–463. https://www-proquest-com.fgul.idm.oclc.org/docview/1674426289?pq-origsite= summon&accountid=10868

xv Beahrs, J.O. (1989). Spontaneous hypnosis in the forensic context. *Bulletiin of the American Academy of Psychiatry Law*, 17(2), 171–181. https://jaapl.org/content/ jaapl/17/2/171.full.pdf

Introduction

Professional first responders never know what to expect when they receive the call to attend to a medical emergency. Upon arriving at the scene, they must quickly determine what is wrong with the patient and quickly address any life-threatening problems. Moreover, it is likely that chaos is all around. The patient may be complaining about their pain or worried about their belongings or pets. Family members or other people at the scene might be getting in the way while trying to comfort the patient or even challenging what the medic is doing. Emergency scenes are often overwhelming and require effective communication skills to coordinate procedures and calm everyone down, preventing negative language that can make the situation worse.

While such scene management skills are developed over time and require the art of being patient with others, most first responders have not been trained in optimal communication skills beyond being told to "calm and reassure" the patient. They do their best to employ the correct medical interventions without awareness of the potential for negative communication that can cause harm to the patient. This book addresses this problem and goes further than just preventing potentially hurtful language. It shows how by recognizing that people in medical emergencies often go into a spontaneous hypnosis state that makes them hyper-suggestible to the directives of a trusted individual. We teach you how to use words to augment standard medical care in ways that recognize this phenomenon. With an understanding of basic hypnotic communication strategies, you can not only calm and reassure but also do much more to alleviate suffering and encourage healing.[1,2]

For way too long, pre-hospital emergency workers have used inappropriate words at the emergency scene. This includes harsh or even rude language or aggressive interrogations. When this happens, it is usually not intentional. Rather, it stems from the first responder's own anxieties and fears about being effective and dealing with the trauma at hand, perhaps only minutes after having just attended a previous one. Just managing traffic with sirens blasting and trying to find the location of the emergency as quickly as possible creates enough stress to cause language to be abrupt at the least. Add to this the knowledge that the

DOI: 10.4324/9781003430261-1

first responder knows they will be accountable for whatever happens, and one can appreciate even with knowledge of correct language use, communication can be inappropriate and potentially harmful.

But what is an appropriate conversation? Why do words have such power? What potential is there for the positive influence of words? How can we learn to project calmness and reassurance in the face of frightening events and life-threatening injuries or illnesses?

In short, what is the most effective way to communicate with a person in trauma? This book answers these questions and presents communication strategies that can tap the inner resources of a patient. It is based on research that continues to show that certain kinds of verbal and nonverbal communication with people under stress can influence virtually every nervous system function and its result—from bleeding and blood pressure to inflammation and immune response. It is also based on evidence indicating that proper communication can increase the effectiveness of standard medical treatment. It may be "the most effective treatment you have yet to prescribe" (or use).[3]

This book presents guidelines, strategies, and techniques that can be used in the field, not only to prevent what but also to enhance a patient's natural survival and healing capabilities. Theoretically, doing this work can even have a long-term positive effect. When negative emotions and inappropriate interpretations become deeply rooted in a medical emergency patient, they can remain self-defeating for many years, even after physical recovery. Many post-trauma stress disorders have been traced back to less-than-optimal communication at the emergency scene. Using proper communication techniques can not only enhance recovery immediately after trauma but also prevent future anxiety syndromes.

Thus, you are about to expand the boundaries of primary care and take advantage of the mind-body connection. This calls for assuming that our thoughts, beliefs, and attitudes send messages to every part of our body that either can encourage or discourage optimal functioning. When we are frightened, confused, or seriously injured or ill, our thoughts are often dependent on what is told to us by confident voices. When these voices know how to direct positive responses, they can be lifesaving, especially when the communication occurs within the first-hour post-trauma, before stressful reactions become more deeply rooted. This text will help you become that confident, knowing voice so that your words can augment whatever standard emergency medical care approaches you may have learned. They will not replace and should not interrupt such care, but are vital nonetheless. When you communicate with a person dealing with a medical emergency, your words touch the tip of an iceberg. Beneath the surface, numerous associations and responses can be set in motion. Often, these occur at the unconscious (subconscious) level. When they do, every word, phrase, sentence, pause, voice inflection, and gesture can initiate automatic psychophysiological effects. As a result, most patients experiencing a medical emergency are incredibly vulnerable because they are thrust into a psychological state that predisposes them to hypnosis. The patient who experiences this phenomenon may be around people who hurt or heal them just based on how they communicate.

This sensitive receptivity to words and gestures is the most acute during the first hour of the medical emergency or trauma. If after this amount of time external communication is not received, people faced with the emergency begin to rely on their own internal communication. Using past experience or learned associations, patients begin to interpret their predicament and respond to it accordingly. During the first hour or so, however, it appears that injured, frightened or confused people focus their entire attention on trying to understand the situation by waiting for appropriate directions. This may be why people tend to freeze during surprising or sudden emergencies until someone finally shouts, "Don't just stand there, call 911!"

Unfortunately, the past associations of most people are not optimal for coping with medical emergencies. Instead, they create added stress. It is generally agreed that mental stress contributes significantly to the majority of medical problems. Medical emergencies are no exception. Stress impairs the immune system and weakens organs and glands.[4] When combined with physical injury, it impedes recovery. The art of effective communication with persons in trauma thus relates to using words and gestures to minimize negative stress and maximize healing processes. To do this calls for an understanding that during the first hour of trauma, most people are in a hyper-suggestible state of consciousness. In effect, they are in a state of spontaneous hypnosis. Thus, words can direct patients to control to some degree their own optimal nervous system functioning in ways that can activate self-healing mechanisms such as reducing pain sensation and blood pressure.

In the chapters that follow, we show you how to understand and utilize such words that take advantage of the spontaneous hypnotic state you can assume most emergency victims enter. This makes them receptive to appropriate communication from a trusted first responder. To help with learning and remembering how to project such trust and how to use hypnotic language, we use the mnemonic **C R E D I B L E** (representing the words Confidence, Rapport, Expectation, Directives, Images, Believability, Literalness, and Enthusiasm). Each chapter addresses a part of this mnemonic.

Part I teaches ways to increase the believability of what you say to the patient. Chapter 1 offers information that illustrates the effectiveness of this kind of communication. Chapter 2 teaches you how to project Confidence at the emergency scene. Chapter 3 shows you how to gain and maintain proper Rapport with the person in trauma. Chapter 4 describes how to build the patient's Expectations for a positive, hopeful future.

Part II offers guidelines for giving the emergency patient directives that can tap one's own powerful coping abilities. Chapter 5 begins by teaching specific guidelines for such communication. Chapters 6 through 9 use the C R E D **I B L E** mnemonic's suffix (**I**mages, **B**elievability, **L**iteralness, and **E**nthusiasm) to present basic rules and illustrations that will help assure that directives to the patient will be successful. Chapters 10 through 17 discuss particular emergency situations and offer phrasing examples that use the techniques described in earlier chapters. (The examples are based on actual case studies where they were used effectively. It is suggested that they be memorized, then modified to suit unique situations and communication styles.) Chapter 18 gives information on the use of self-talk and belief systems that can help you survive a personal trauma. Finally, Chapter 19 tells how the same principles of language and thoughts that can dramatically influence human biology can contribute to the saving of the planet.

Legal and Ethical Considerations

Although some states have laws about practicing hypnotherapy, they should not apply to patient communication skills that recognize and use language to medical emergency patients who are probably in a state of spontaneous hypnosis. The medic is simply avoiding words that can do harm while giving directives that can calm and potentially heal. To ask if it is legal or ethical to use words accordingly would require one to ask if it might be illegal and unethical to say the wrong things. Consider this hypothetical situation. Two paramedics respond to an emergency call for help. When they arrive on the scene, they find a 32-year-old female complaining of nausea and acute back pain. She states that she has been passing blood in her urine for several hours. The paramedics follow standard care protocols and proceed to transport the patient to the hospital in the ambulance. Riding in the back of the ambulance with the patient along with one of the paramedics is the woman's five-year-old daughter. On the way to the hospital, the patient's vital signs begin to diminish. Seriously concerned and emotionally distraught by the tears of the little girl, the paramedic in the back says to the paramedic who is driving, "Hurry up John, she won't make it if we don't get there soon." The woman is dead on arrival and cardiopulmonary resuscitation (CPR) efforts are unsuccessful. Shortly after, the woman's family learns from his daughter that one of the paramedics said, "she won't make it." Is the county or the paramedic liable for negligence? Probably not. Did the paramedic help the situation? Definitely not. Might the woman have lived if he had not said the words? It is possible based on what we know about the power of words.

The point is that although we state here and throughout the book that words spoken with hypnosis in mind should be used only as an adjunct to standard medical care, learning how to positively phrase healing suggestions is a vital opportunity to help medical emergency patients.

In his book, *Selective Awareness*, Peter Mutke, M.D., describes several cases of iatrogenic communication. (Iatrogenic is defined in Tabor's *Cyclopedic Medical Dictionary* as "an abnormal mental or physical condition induced in a patient by effects of treatment by a physician or surgeon. The term implies that such effects could have been avoided by proper and judicious care on the part of the physician.") The cases Dr. Mutke presents involve paramedical personnel and nurses, as well as physicians. In each situation, statements made by rescuers either slowed down or stopped the self-corrective abilities of the patients. The iatrogenic statements were sometimes no more than a careless remark that was overheard or misinterpreted by the patient. In all cases, however, the result was a limited and pessimistic outlook for the recovery of health.

In most instances, the legal principle that all first responders must abide by when performing a rescue is the principle of nonmaleficence. This simply means "to do no further harm." One exception to this principle occurs when a reasonable person could not have foreseen the consequences of a particular action. Similarly, in the United States, under Good Samaritan laws, rescuers may not be liable "for acts done in good faith." Whether a statement such as "That's the worst hip fracture I've ever seen" or "I don't think this guy is gonna make it" would be construed as reasonable or in good faith would pose an interesting question. Thus, the mandate to "avoid inappropriate conversation at the scene of an emergency" may carry with it some legal, if not moral, accountability. But what about legal and moral issues that relate to using positive communication strategies to enhance recovery from medical emergencies? If you are able to direct a patient to stop their bleeding with your words and manner, are you stepping outside your boundary?

The "Code of Ethics for Emergency Medical Technicians" adopted by the National Association of Emergency Medical Technicians in 1979 suggests that the answer to this question would be no. It states that the basic responsibility of the EMT is to "conserve life, to alleviate suffering and to promote health." Since there is no injunction against speaking to a patient with confidence, using effective communication skills to offer hope, or suggesting the action of natural healing mechanisms, it would be difficult to imagine a case where you would be liable for directing a patient to stop bleeding, whether or not it worked, *as long as it did not interfere with the standard procedures for treatment.*

Countertransference

First responders and emergency medical services (EMS) personnel who utilize this book's approach to patient care will possibly risk *countertransference* more than those who continue to exclusively use a mechanistic, technical approach. Recognizing this possibility and taking appropriate remedial action will help prevent any lasting repercussions.

Countertransference refers to symptoms or stress passed on from patient to rescuer as a result of shared involvement in the treatment efforts. When the first responder, EMT, or paramedic enters into the kind of rapport with a patient required to achieve the results that have been described, unconscious emotional contents can be transferred back and forth between two individuals. This transference can touch unresolved or sensitive issues in the rescuer's unconscious that relate to fear of death, loss of relationships, parental control or abandonment, vulnerability, and so on. Occasionally, physical symptoms similar to those manifested by the patient can be temporarily exhibited by the rescuer.

The first step in preventing or removing countertransference hazards is to allow for full emotional involvement with the patient while still maintaining professional rapport. Do not allow any fears of countertransference or unconscious impulses to cause you to repress the interconnected consciousness that you share with the patient.

The second step is to attempt to access and ventilate feelings and thoughts after the emergency incident is over. This can be done with coworkers or a professional counselor, anyone who has been trained to take this post-trauma exercise seriously.

The third step is to maintain a well-balanced lifestyle in general. Sufficient physical exercise to release physical tension and strengthen cardiovascular systems should be taken regularly. Alcohol usage should be limited and mind-altering drugs should be avoided entirely. Hobbies and interests unrelated to the emergency rescue field should also be developed.

And finally, countertransference should be viewed philosophically as an opportunity to realize that we all do indeed share in one another's thoughts and emotions to some degree. We all influence one another with our thoughts. With this understanding, learned over and over again from the countertransference phenomenon, we may better be able to perceive our connection with all things. The biological stress response was designed to prevent injury by mobilizing fight or flight capabilities. For example, the immune and digestive systems are shut down. Blood pressure is increased. After the injury, when the danger of further trauma is passed, this response is no longer helpful. Psychological concerns, however, are nonetheless interpreted by the nervous system as another physical threat requiring fight or flight.

With the aforementioned ideas in the Preface and Introduction in mind, you may be ready to start learning how to employ positive hypnotic language while treating the injured or ill victim with standard medical care. It is important to understand what we have presented so far in order for you to give sufficient credibility to the concept of emergency hypnosis to be motivated to use this approach and to be effective when you do.

Notes

1 Peebles-Kleiger, M.J. (2000). The use of hypnosis in emergency medicine. *Emergency Medicine Clinics of North America*, 18(2), 327–338. https://pubmed.ncbi.nlm.nih.gov/10767888/

2 Oakley, D., & Halligan, P. (2013). Hypnotic suggestion: Opportunities for cognitive neuroscience. *Nature Reviews Neuroscience*, 14, 565–576. https://doi.org/10.1038/nrn3538

3 Kittle, J., & Spiegel, D. (2021). Hypnosis: The most effective treatment you have yet to prescribe. *The American Journal of Medicine*, 134(3), 304–305.

4 Drigas, A., & Mitsea, E. (2021). Metacognition, stress-relaxation balance & related hormones. *International Journal of Recent Contributions from Engineering, Science, and IT*, 9(1), 4–16.

Part I

1 Credibility

The objective of this chapter is to help with understanding the potential of proper communication with the person in trauma and convey sufficient credibility and confidence to the patient. Before words can have a profound effect on someone, they must also be believed sufficiently by the patient for the hypnosis to take effect. It is from this sense of credibility that we are motivated to listen and react. Remember, people become hyper-suggestible to the directives of a perceived trusted authority figure. Imagine if you were seated at a cafe and a firefighter walked in and confidently declared "I want everyone to stand up now and walk without hesitation to the exit because there is a fire next door about to jump over to this building." Would you be more likely to follow the directive decisively than if a nine-year-old came in and said there is a fire next door. "You better all get out of here?" If you had high blood pressure and a paramedic confidently told you to take a deep breath, relax into it and imagine your blood vessels expanding and flowing blood as I pump the BP cuff up on your arm, the evidence has shown that blood pressure may well go down. Giving such a directive without offering confidence and credibility would likely fail.

An extreme example of the potential power of words spoken confidently to a person in hypnosis might be voodoo-induced death. This has actually been studied. In 1942, Walter Cannon described such "death by fright" incidents as relating to an absolute belief the power of a Medicine Person to do this and caused a "lasting and intense action of the sympathetic-adrenal system".[1] Curt Richter reported on a series of experiments about Cannon's views that revealed sympathetic and parasympathetic effects result in bradycardia developed prior to death.[2] This hints at the possibility of incorrect words spoken to a frightened highly suggestive patient, such as the example we gave in the Introduction. Although it is very unlikely that you or I would be affected by such a directive, people who grow up *believing* in the ability (giving credibility) can die when they and their community watch the medicine person stick a needle in the heart of a doll representing the victim.

Of course, a first responder saying inadvertently to a fellow medic loud enough for the patient to hear, "I don't think this person is going to survive" is a long

DOI: 10.4324/9781003430261-3

way from the intentional voodoo curse. However, the results may be similar. This underscores the reasons the American Academic of Orthopedic Surgeons warns in its emergency care book that words can cause untold harm, as previously noted. Belief in the images words can produce in the brain can have significant positive or negative effects on neurotransmitters when a person is in the hypnotic state of receptivity. However, one does not even have to be in hypnosis for such beliefs to occur. For many years, it was believed that no one would ever break the four-minute mile. Though many coaches tried to persuade athletes to run faster and faster, the barrier remained unbroken until one day Jim Ryun managed the "impossible." Within six months, high school and college runners from around the world began running the distance in less than four minutes. Coaches obviously were using the same verbal persuasion as before, but now their words had a sense of credibility.

Such beliefs can relate to the use of placebos in medical experiments, spontaneous remission of incurable diseases, commercial advertising, religious healing, and host of therapies that have sufficient "credibility" in the mind of someone using them. If a first responder is to be successful when using the directives presented in this text, recognizing the power of hypnotic communication is crucial. Not only will it help prevent saying something potentially harmful but also it can inspire using positive language to induce nervous system responses in the patient that can lead to survival, pain reduction, and healing. With this in mind, we finish this chapter with some more ideas about the power of words as a rapid healing force.

Healing with Words: A Historical Perspective

Before the language of words, humans thought only with images. The earliest humans painted the visions of their beliefs on cave walls to share with others in the community and to give them an external reality. Their thoughts and emotions were images in their minds and could only be expressed through gestures of art, dance, and other ritualistic practices. The individuals most expressive in these things became the healers of society. Their ability to get the sick and injured to associate healthful images with ritual worked often enough for others to gain trust for them. Healing shamans were common in preliterate cultures.

As verbal communication developed, words came to function as labels. With labels, objects and experiences could be analyzed and categorized. For example, they were good or bad, safe or dangerous, and threatening or nonthreatening. As the process has evolved, however, there have been errors in judgment, conflicting meanings, and rampant generalizing. New or unlabeled experiences became associated with the categories filed in each person's brain. For example, the experience described by the word *adventure* could be associated with danger, opportunity, challenge, fun, and discomfort. Thus, the reaction to the word would depend on the particular association.

In this book, you will learn to "unlabel" when communicating directly with an emergency patient. For example, if a patient claims to be an asthmatic or a diabetic, it is helpful to reframe that person's perspective of themself as someone who has a history of suffering from diabetic or asthmatic symptoms. When a paramedic or an emergency medical technician (EMT) asks a patient questions, they are not only trying to find out what is wrong but are also trying to find out what symptoms match a known disease. When an illness is viewed as a process rather than as a part of the person, it is easier to treat or cure it.

As language evolved in this way, medical cures became associated with certain illnesses or injuries. Until relatively recent times, most of the medications that were successful in treating a variety of ills were either pharmacologically inert or based on marginal research. This *placebo effect*, however, has continued to play a significant role in the effect of modern medication. In fact, numerous studies have revealed that the effectiveness of most major medications is due to the placebo effect. In other words, a high percentage of people given placebos obtain identical results as those given the actual medication. A study led by Kaptchuk and published in *Science Translational Medicine* explored this by testing how people reacted to migraine pain medication. One group took a migraine drug labeled with the drug's name, another took a placebo labeled "placebo," and a third group took nothing. The researchers discovered that the placebo was 50 percent as effective as the real drug to reduce pain after a migraine attack.[3]

The placebo effect demonstrates that what we believe and have faith or trust in can affect the nervous system more effectively than drugs. In one study, belief even reversed the chemical effect of medication. Patients suffering from chronic nausea were given a "new medicine" to stop their vomiting, and it worked. The medicine, however, was ipecac, a substance that normally induces vomiting. This was first reported in the seminal work of Stewart Wolf:

> Although ipecac is commonly used to induce vomiting when toxic substances have been swallowed, Wolf misinformed his patient that it was a medicine which would alleviate her nausea. Prior to taking ipecac, the patient displayed an absence of gastric contractions. Within 20 minutes of ingesting the drug, normal gastric contractions resumed and the nausea ended.[4]

It may be that the so-called placebo effect is also at work for some surgical procedures. In the 1960s, a physician named Beecher published the results of an experiment relating to the treatment of angina.[5] At that time, an operation referred to as the internal mammary ligation procedure was used to treat angina pain. Internal mammary arteries were tied off to increase blood flow through the coronary artery. The procedure resulted in objectively measured improvements in 98 percent of the cases. Beecher matched patients for age, sex, and duration of illness and performed the operation on half of them. On the other half, he performed a mock operation whereby he prepared them for surgery, anesthetized them, and made an incision in the chest. No further intervention was done with these patients, however. The incision was simply made, then sutured. After recovery, the benefits of the real operation and the mock operation were identical on all objective and subjective measurements, including stress testing.

There have been numerous other studies demonstrating the influence of belief or expectations on surgical procedures. Many have been described in the books listed in the bibliography. Such studies have been reported officially since the advent of modern surgical procedures. For example, in the nineteenth century, several physicians published reports on "painless" surgical operations without the usual high rate of infection and mortality that occurred before the use of chemical anesthesia and sterilization.

The most famous was Dr. James Esdaile, who performed hundreds of such operations while working in India. Most of Dr. Esdaile's patients were natives who believed in the Indian practice of *jar-phoonk*. Jar-phoonk was a ritual that native healers performed on the sick. It consisted of rhythmical stroking and blowing air on a patient until they became relaxed and seemingly distracted from their pain.

Dr. Esdaile's work was neither researched nor welcomed by the medical profession in general. In fact, his practices were treated with much hostility and ridiculed by his colleagues. This happened because the orthodox physicians were then trying to free themselves from past connections with magic and religious healing. Struggling to establish an image for themselves as being strictly scientific, the medical profession continued to separate itself from mind-body research.

The Kansas Experiment

This effort to separate traditional physical medicine from psychology has carried over into the field of medicine as well. In 1976, M. Erik Wright, M.D., Ph.D., an internationally renowned psychologist and psychiatrist, conducted a pioneering research project at an emergency hospital in Kansas. He trained three groups of ambulance technicians to carefully follow several simple communication procedures with emergency patients. First, they were to remove the patient from the crowd as soon as possible to prevent the patient from hearing crowd noise. Second, they were to recite a memorized paragraph designed to calm and reassure the patient and encourage the patient's body systems to work toward survival. The words were to be repeated in a low tone with the paramedic's mouth close to the patient's ear. This was to be done whether or not the patient was unconscious and, of course, like all the procedures in this book, was to be used as an adjunct to standard medical care. Third, no other conversation between the paramedics that could be construed as negative or unrelated to the patient could occur.

The demonstration experiment lasted six months. Treatment outcomes of the patients attended to by the trained paramedics were compared with those of control groups who went about business as usual and who were not so instructed. The results were significant: *The experimental group of patients had more people survive the trip to the Hospital and had shorter hospital stays and quicker recovery rates.*

In spite of the remarkable findings of this landmark demonstration, the training program was dropped by the hospital administration when the research funds were exhausted. In a presentation before a group of physicians attending an American Society of Clinical Hypnosis Conference, Dr. Wright described the research and his dismay that the training was not continued. As mentioned in the Introduction, until recently the reluctance of the medical field's gatekeepers to allow other than physicians to use hypnosis was common. Wright's speech testifies to the importance of proper communication with the emergency patient. His speech is quoted, as follows, in its entirety.

This study had to do with the training of ambulance attendants who go to a traumatic situation to pick up individuals in various states of tremendous trauma to the body, varying from car accidents, overdoses of drugs, and traumatic events of various kinds, including those not as severely traumatized but nevertheless who cannot bring themselves to the emergency room or hospital situation. These individuals, through the impact of an emergency environment, began to have the terror of survival, the fear of whether or not there is going to be the next moment. And there has been a radical alteration of the life space. The psychological life space has suddenly shrunk so that most of the visually important factors in their life are inconsequential.

Rather, the immediate awareness of the body and the surrounding environment have closed down and the narrowing of the total psychological functioning has occurred so that there is an acute responsiveness in some areas and a lack of awareness in others. This, I think, is important to emphasize besides the physiological mobilization that has been energized by the trauma. Even shock can be considered a radical mobilization of the body to preserve essential life functions by placing the body in a condition of minimum functioning in order to sustain survival for a given moment. Given these circumstances and some of the interesting observations of David Cheek and others, we develop the thesis that in such situations, the person's usual critical responsiveness to the environment has been altered so that whatever stimuli do reach—whatever language is comprehended, whatever communications are received—are often subject to a literal translation and can either aggravate or support the life systems that are hanging on.

In the experiment, the ambulance attendants were taught a general statement they were to tell the patient as soon as they reached the patient:

The worst is over. We are taking you to the hospital. Everything is being made ready. Let your body concentrate on repairing itself and feeling secure. Let your heart, your blood vessels, everything, bring themselves into a state of preserving your life. Bleed just enough so as to cleanse the wound, and let the blood vessels close down so that your life is preserved. Your body weight, your body heat, everything, is being maintained. Things are being made ready at the hospital for you. We're getting there as quickly and safely as possible. You are now in a safe position. The worst is over.

This kind of rhetoric was repeated in a low-key voice with the mouth of the attendant close to the patients, whether they were stuporous, conscious, or unconscious.

The medics were also advised to get quickly away from the crowd—with all their comments, like "Hey, is that guy gonna die?" or "Gee, that's a mess," and all of the interventions of police and others who are so eager to see the "mess" come to a dramatic end. It's incredible, the language a patient is subject to at the emergency scene.

Now, this emphasis on the messages being fed in also helped keep the attendants from talking between themselves, because they can be the most traumatizing of the patient's exposure to language as they drive the patient back to the hospital. They might say, "Man, that's a goner back there," and other things that are said with their focus upon concerns like will they get back in time to catch the last game of the world series and so on. They picked the patient up, put him in a splint, set the IV bottle going with a transfusion, and have called in ahead, and that's it.

The training program taught the attendants to be consciously aware of their responsibility. It seems absurd to find that such a relatively minor intervention—at least in the demonstration experiences, which lasted six months, comparing the random patients that were picked up by the experimental crews (there were three crews) with the patients that were picked up by the nontrained control crews could make such a difference in, first, the number who were not dead on arrival but who survived the trip, those who were sustained and able to be treated, and those who had a quicker recovery rate. Now the fact that this demonstration was statistically valid doesn't mean that the process of training was adopted, because once the demonstration funds ran out, nothing else was done about it. That's quite independent. But from the point of view of a demonstration of a radical shift, which look into account that in a state of severe traumatization, there is still (as long as life persists) a communication system. There is still a focus of attention where the critical state of the patient has caused an uncritical acceptance of options. The support framework of language becomes a significant contributor to the healthcare management of the individual. It is so absurdly simple that you become, at least I become, terribly distressed, because you can't budge administrative organizations to initiate this kind of processing. During the training, the [paramedics] themselves become the proselytizers and we had difficulty in keeping them from spoiling the experiment and teaching the others. So, the environment of treatment begins with the first initial contact between any of the medical viable personnel to the very last terminal relationship when the patient leaves the hospital. We need to understand the need for a structure of language which is supportive and recognizes the translation of comments.[6]

How Words Influence Healing

When we see with our eyes, what we ultimately perceive relates to a photochemical reaction that triggers nerve impulses conducted to the brain's cerebral cortex. This area of the brain decodes the impulses via image responsive chemicals that create our perception. Whether or not the images are meaningful is determined by learned experience. All we need in order to experience an image and an associated perception is for the appropriate neuronal pathways to fire. It does not matter whether they fire because of stimulation to the retina or other sense organs, or because of an internal image, such as dream, imagination, or memory image.

Medical science has been aware of this fact since the 1920s, when American physician and physiologist Dr. Edmund Jacobson did experiments proving that, when people imagined themselves involved in an action like running or swimming, the muscles in their body associated with that action contracted in amounts that could be measured with special equipment. Further research has shown that virtually every cell in the body can be influenced by images held in the mind's eye. Through the pathways between the cerebral cortex, where images are stored, and the automatic nervous system, such images can control:

sweating
blood pressure
blood vessel expansion and contraction
flushing
goose pimpling
pain response
heart rate and force of contraction
respiratory rate
dryness of mouth
immune response
bowel motility
smooth muscle tension
glandular secretions
inflammatory response
blood coagulation
allergic response
rate of healing
dermatitis
emotional reactions
and more.

During times of fear, emotional factors combine with old belief systems to create images that may influence one or more of the above functions negatively. The same factors, however, can make an individual highly receptive toward new directions from someone who is perceived as a trusted leader or authority figure. This process seems to occur in animals as well.[7] Frightened wild animals can be extremely trusting of confident and caring humans, allowing themselves to be handled or cared for. In fact, Four Arrows learned much about spontaneous hypnosis from his work with wild horses,[8] as he mentions in the Preface.

Perhaps this increased receptivity and specific focus involved with hypnotic states of mind is a natural protective mechanism common to all species. In times of confusion, it allows for quick responses to the directions of herd or tribal leaders. If this is a primitive survival function, it makes sense that it is initiated in the limbic system, the oldest part of the brain. The major function of the limbic system is to compare incoming stimuli from the body with instructions programmed by previous experiences. It interacts with the cerebral cortex in analyzing data.

A component of the limbic system is the *amygdala*. Here emotional responses are triggered when incoming stimuli do not fit expected patterns. If something new and unexpected happens, like a medical emergency, it will send out impulses that trigger the release of hormones in an effort to prepare the body for fight or flight. Unfortunately, most of the programming of past experiences that directs the activity of the amygdala consists of old patterns that were programmed during infancy and early childhood when we were not sufficiently conscious to clearly evaluate the addictions of our parents, teachers, and others. Because these instructions still reside in our biocomputers, in most emergency situations (in our culture) we end up doing that which violates our first survival interests. In most cases, neither fight nor flight is an appropriate reaction.

Fortunately, fear, stress, and confusion also increase the potential for adaptation by increasing activity in the brain's image center. Many researchers believe that such image-making activity occurs in the right hemisphere of the brain. Julian Jaynes, author of *The Origin of Consciousness in the Breakdown of the Bicameral Mind*, suggests that right-brained, holographic activity is precipitated by stress. He hypothesized that the more acute the suffering, the stronger the stimulus compensating image production by the right hemisphere. He did not, however, talk about the effect of words, whether from ones own mind or from a first responder on the scene during the suffering, to trigger positive images.

It is known that the image-responsive chemicals in the right brain somehow trigger the secretion of hormones, including neurohormones, that control the pituitary and endocrine systems, adrenalin, noradrenalin, and endorphins. Ultimately, these hormones and others are involved in the regulation of the sympathetic and parasympathetic nervous system. Language centers in the left brain provide a mode of access for the description and interpretation of images. However, the specific relationship between words and images is not understood. Words not only describe images but also create them.

We do know, however, that there are at least three times when image-responsive centers in the brain become active enough to affect physiological processes that can enhance recovery from medical emergencies. These three times are as follows:

1 Following the acceptance of a belief. Images follow beliefs. When belief is formed, the mind begins to accept images that relate to it. Placebos are an example of this. The more a patient believes in the rescuer, the more likely the rescuer's words will cause the creation of effective healing images.
2 While involved in passive concentration. Image activity also increases when active, analytical thinking slows down and is replaced with focused attention. This focus is fundamental to things such as hypnosis, self-hypnosis, biofeedback, meditation, yoga, autogenics, visualization, and Zen. This kind of concentration requires training and practice.
3 During periods of emotional excitement, emotions prepare the body to defend itself against harm. Fear increases the ability to run away, while anger increases aggressive capabilities. As we have mentioned, however, when neither fight nor flight is appropriate, the emotional state opens up receptivity to the suggestions of a trusted authority figure. This partially explains the power a charismatic, trusted individual can have over people during times of stress. History is full of illustrations where such leaders have persuaded people to do remarkable things, good or bad.

Body Language

It is important to remember, as you study the communication strategies in the next few chapters, that the delivery of words is as important as the words alone while attempting to influence the patient's images. Dr. Noel Burch is coauthor (with Dr. Thomas Gordon) of *Teacher Effectiveness Training.*[9] Using Dr. Ray L. Birdwhistell's research From the University of Pennsylvania, Dr. Burch says that, when a person is communicating, 70 percent of his message is sent by body language, 23 percent by the tone or inflection of voice, and only 7 percent by the words that are used.[10,11] Of course, this research was not done with frightened emergency patients, who often cannot see their rescuers clearly during rescue operations. If it had been, it is likely that tone or inflection would have been the most significant. In any case, the importance of nonverbal communication cannot be overstated. These nonverbal expressions are often more reliable indicators of our true feelings than words. If you want to actually connect with someone, you will need to express that through your body language. To do this you might lean in when they are talking, make eye contact (unless you know they come from a culture where this is not a good thing), genuinely connect with them with sincerity and caring, and be aware of their body language messages.

Nonverbal expressions are part of the foundation to building a healing relationship with the emergency patient during the short time you may have with them. (Remember, after an hour hypnotic language is less effective because the patient's own belief systems will have taken over internal self-hypnotic responses, for better or worse.) Many books have been written on the subject of body language, but all you need to know as a first responder is to be confident, sincere, and caring and you will convey this automatically.

True or False?

1 Protective mechanisms in the body can overreact to injury and illness.
2 Words and images can influence autonomic nervous system functions.
3 Dr. Wright's Kansas experiment showed that the words spoken by paramedics had no significant effect on treatment outcome.
4 Fear increases receptivity to the directions of a trusted authority figure.
5 Body language is not as important as words.

Notes

1 Samuels, N. (2007). Voodoo death reisted: The modern lessons of neurocardiology. *Cleveland Clinic Journal of Medicine.* https://www.semanticscholar.org/paper/
   'Voodoo'-death-revisited%3A-the-modern-lessons-of-Samuels/715fbad0bbe7ea2f9
   78baee742c8f57507444c98
2 Ibid.
3 Harvard Health (December, 2021). The power of the placebo effect. health.harvard.
   edu/mental-health/the-power-of-the-placebo-effect
4 Kirsch, I. (2008). Challenging received wisdom: Antidepressants and the placebo effect. *Mcgill Journal of Medicine,* 11(2), 219–222. https://www.ncbi.nlm.nih.gov/
   pmc/articles/PMC2582668/
5 Beecher, H.D. (1961 July). Surgery as placebo. A quantitative study. *Journal of the American Medical Association (JAMA),* 176, 1102–1107. https://pubmed.ncbi.nlm.
   nih.gov/13688614/
6 From Wright's presentation in 1977 at the American Society of Clinical Hypnosis conference. Personal papers of M. Erik wright. University of Kansas, Kenneth Spencer Research Library. https://archives.lib.ku.edu/repositories/3/resources/137
7 Gilman, T.T., & Marcuse, F.L. (1949). Animal hypnosis. *Psychological Bulletin,* 46(2), 151–165. https://doi.org/10.1037/h0060434
8 See Four Arrows wild horse hypnotist. *Youtube* https://www.youtube.com/
   watch?v=vxzAm08731c
9 Gordon, T., & Burch, N. (1974). *TET Teacher Effectiveness Training.* David McKay Company.
10 Birdwhistell, R. L. (1952). *Introduction to Kinesics: An Annotation System for Analysis of Body Motion and Gesture.* Department of State, Foreign Service Institute.
11 Birdwhistell, R. L. (1970). *Kinesics and Context: Essays on Body Motion Communication.* University of Pennsylvania Press.

2   Confidence

The main objective of this chapter is to teach how to project confidence at the emergency scene. The word confidence represents the first letter of the mnemonic **C**REDIBLE and stands as an important aspect of hypnotic communication. If a first responder does not speak like they are in control, knowledgeable, and trustworthy, the patient's attention may go elsewhere, and the directives' healing potential may be minimal. Projecting confidence is the first step toward preparing the patient to accept messages that can mobilize health-stabilizing responses. We recommend getting a handle on one's projection of confidence as clarity on the next steps before touching or speaking to the patient.

Sometimes victims of medical emergencies will trust a professional rescuer simply because of the official uniform. However, this is usually not enough. First responders may not always be in uniform. Some injuries prevent a patient from seeing their rescuers. Occasionally a uniform can trigger distrust. Furthermore, a patient may quickly lose confidence in uniformed personnel if their words and manner reflect a lack of confidence.

Guidelines for Projecting Confidence

Develop Authentic Faith in Yourself

To put forth and maintain confidence amidst a crisis, you must have faith in yourself. This means believing in your ability to use your first aid skills and knowledge *as best you can*. Such a belief comes from knowing your strengths, acknowledging your weaknesses (while working to improve them), and going all out to achieve what you can for the patient. Research for my own dissertation research shows that the intuition that comes from experience can often lead to more effective outcomes over a strict memorization of intervention steps.[1] This willingness to face any problem within the range of your capabilities provides the experiences necessary to develop a confident attitude at the emergency scene.

It is important to be realistic about your strengths and weaknesses while developing such a confident belief in your abilities. Every call is different, but

DOI: 10.4324/9781003430261-4

there are common issues one can learn to address without hesitation. If you have a partner that knows a technique better, then let her/him do it and concentrate on the hypnotic language you will need to learn. By the end of this book you will learn the skill yourself. If you try to do more than your abilities allow, attempting to overcompensate for a lack of confidence, you are likely to make mistakes that will decrease your confidence further.

To learn your strengths and weaknesses and develop confidence, make a list of them and determine which ones you can improve. Remember to analyze rather than criticize them. It is useful to discuss how things went after a call to do this. Continual training in medical and rescue procedures is also important, as is having faith in one's equipment.

Finally, using self-hypnosis, both in training/learning and before you communicate with the patient is a powerful way to bring forth an aura of confidence. Practicing self-hypnosis to get good at it will often allow for a quick triggering of the automatic nervous system to turn on positive, confidence-building emotions.

Stay in Top Physical Condition

Physical fitness breeds confidence, whether or not an emergency response requires a strenuous task. Of course, a fit rescuer will have the strength and stamina sometimes necessary. The mere fact of accomplishing a difficult physical action like climbing down a dangerous cliff or carrying someone out of harm's way will go a long way toward building confidence and credibility. Fitness also helps with providing reserves of energy that can help with clear thinking and calm communication with the victim, even after long days and many calls.

Move from Fear to Courage

Fear, apprehension and/or anxiety are reasonable emotions for a first responder to have on the way to, or upon arriving at an unimaginable emergency scene. A degree of fear is appropriate. It can serve as a warning to carefully assess the situation and to act appropriately to avoid danger if possible. Once fear has served this function, however, there is no longer any need to hold on to it. Not turning the fear into courage or a "fearless trust in the universe"[2] Doing so will cause unnecessary stress and will detract from your ability to project confidence to the frightened patient. Using self-hypnosis can also help with this flow from fear to fearlessness.[3]

Besides the fear of physical harm, first responders are often fearful of psychological or "ego" harm. They are afraid to say the wrong thing, to use the incorrect first aid procedure, or to appear foolish while using special communication strategies described in this test. They may also be afraid of legal consequences relative to helping a medical emergency patient if it is necessary to take an unusual risk.

Whatever the particular stimulus for fear, the first step is to keep this emotion in *motion*. This means moving beyond it by realizing the nature of actual risks and probably benefits of any action being considered. This helps break the cycle of fear from increasing illogically. When we stop wrestling with fear and use reason and positive images on behalf of a goal, fear can disappear. If you are still wrestling with it when you speak, the patient will know it. If, instead, you concentrate on the skills, the work, the action, the task, and the needs of the patient, new positive emotions will follow the nature of your concentration, and confidence emerges.

It is important to be aware of the difference between fear and arousal, though the physiological responses are similar. It is natural to have an increase in adrenalin when involved in emergency rescue and care. An increased arousal level by rescue personnel must be controlled so the patient does not become afraid or lose confidence. (Remember, in the mnemonic, CREDIBLE, the "E" refers to just the right amount of enthusiasm.)

Monitor Emotional Reactions

To maintain the positive transference of confidence that is fundamental to the optimal effect of words or treatment outcome, the first-aider must constantly be aware of one's own emotional reactions. Many emergency scenes will present numerous factors that could easily trigger such emotions as anger, disgust, hate, horror, or sadness. The EMT, paramedic, or citizen first responder, must learn to quickly identify and move beyond negative emotions so they do not disrupt confident communication.

A number of professional first responders have learned to utilize appropriate humor to overcome fear. Although humor might be used inappropriately to mask fear or may be in bad taste or upsetting for a patient, used in the right way it can be a powerful force of healing. We talk more about the use of humor in a later chapter.

Whether reasoning, self-hypnosis, or humor can result in the victim having confidence in the rescuer, one should not expect to be able to completely transcend all emotions at the scene of an emergency. To avoid post-traumatic stress after witnessing suffering and death all that might accompany it, such as a child crying for their dead or dying mother, monitoring emotions via ventilating dialogue with a trained mediator or psychologist as soon after the incident as possible. It might be best if your team of first responders is trained in such post-intervention work.

Focus on the Patient—Not Yourself

Perhaps the best way to project confidence at the emergency scene is to focus on the patient and not yourself. In all forms of effective communication, from writing to public speaking, a basic rule is that the speaker thinks of the audience's needs, not their own. When using the techniques and strategies presented in this book to develop rapport, build expectations, and give powerful healing directives, sincere concern for the patient must far outweigh ego considerations. If you worry about how you are going to sound, how you will appear in the eyes of others, or whether or not you will be successful, the chances are that you will not convey sufficient confidence to the patient. Remember that emergency patients become highly aware of their surroundings and will be able to tune in to the degree of sincerity being expressed by those around them. Your personal needs as a rescuer should not be the focus when you are providing patient care. For example, mentioning that you are tired or hungry shows that you are not focused on the priority patient and priority emergency.

Control Your Body Language

In addition to verbal language, a patient perceives messages from nonverbal, intraverbal, and extraverbal signals. Although this occurs during normal communication, the alternative state of consciousness of a frightened emergency patient creates an intensified focus of attention. As a result, such an individual is quick to perceive subtleties of communication that may not be obvious to you. Thus, take care to control the following:

- Nonverbal gestures such as facial expressions, shoulder shrugs, clenched fists, and so on.
- Intraverbal intonations of words. This relates to the emphasis placed on certain words. For example, there is a difference between saying, "We're going to get you *out* of there," and "We're *going* to get you out of there." The former infers a sense of urgency about getting the patient out, which could be a frightening perception to them. The second emphasizes a sense of confidence that there is no doubt the patient is *going* to be extricated.
- Extraverbal implications of words and gestures. Certain dialogues can have tacit meanings that could cause resistance. For example, "Why don't you lie down?" tacitly implies a criticism that might be interpreted, "You fool—why are you standing up?" A better phrase would be, "Would you be more comfortable lying down?"

Frequently a first responder manages to speak with confidence but inadvertently reveals concern, worry, or fear to the patient with their body language. Since most first responders are going to have such thoughts in many instances, it is important to learn how to prevent this unintentional communication.

Actors, courtroom lawyers, diplomats, negotiators, and sales people have all learned both to control their own nonverbal cues and to read them in others. They have learned this with training and practice in voice tone and inflection as well as in control of facial expression, use of hands, posture, and so on. A good way to develop this control is with simulation and feedback sessions. Simulate an emergency situation with a pretend patient and observer. Administer first aid and communicate using the guidelines and scripts contained in this text. Although it will be difficult to reproduce the anxieties and concerns of an actual emergency, try your best to get into the role. A degree of performance anxiety will also help challenge your confidence. The job of the observer is to note the ways in which you convey a lack of confidence. Note the appropriate criticisms, and practice again with different movements, postures, and voice tones until you are able to hide any cues that might convey anxiety or lack of confidence.

Develop a Good Relaxation Response

The ability to project confidence is also related to the ability to relax. Practice makes perfect with this ability as well as practicing appropriate nonverbal communication. Whatever one's profession, learning to quiet ourselves and get in touch with the inner, subtle self through meditation of some form contributes to more relaxed reactions. We recommend at least 15–30 minutes or more using some form of relaxation each day. A variety of alternatives exist, such as autogenic training, Transcendental Meditation, Tai Chi, and yoga. The technique developed by Dr. Edmund Jacobson in the 1920s is also an excellent method.[4] This simply involves making yourself comfortable in an area where you are not likely to be disturbed. Then, beginning with the feet and working up the body to the face and scalp, tighten the muscles, then relax them until the entire body is in a state of relaxation. As you become accustomed to the type of relaxation response you choose, the state of relaxation will occur more and more rapidly until you can enter it spontaneously, even at an emergency scene. Although your arousal level will maintain sufficient adrenalin to help you perform, the ability to relax will help you calm and reassure the patient.

Another way to relax is to be "in the now" as opposed to worrying about past events, things happening in your home or social life, or something that relates to the future. Being in the now is a proven psychological technique for destressing.

Rehearse Your Techniques and Mindset

Once you have developed your own style of communication, perhaps utilizing and modifying the scripts and guidelines presented later, you can practice them like an actor memorizing lines.

This includes both active practices, as in a simulation, mental rehearsal, visualizing the steps, and self-hypnosis, where you visualize yourself when in a meditative or light trance-state. Although each actual emergency situation will be unique, your confidence, intuition and training will come together in optional ways when you visualize emergency medical techniques and the mindset and words you will use at the emergency scene.

Exercises

1 Make a list of your strengths and weaknesses as related to medical emergency responses and skills. Then work on strengthening your weaknesses.
2 Describe a situation or two where a physically fit rescuer would be better prepared to handle an emergency than would be a physically unfit one.
3 Explain the difference between verbal, extraverbal, intraverbal, and nonverbal signals.
4 Describe the Jacobsonian relaxation response.
5 What are examples of how a first responder might mentally be in the future or past during a rescue, rather than in the present?

Notes

1 Duffee, B. (2022). *High-stress high-consequence emergency medical decision making: Paramedics seeking a differential diagnosis.* (Doctoral Dissertation, Fielding Graduate University). Available from ProQuest Dissertations & Theses Global. https://www.proquest.com/docview/2718154892
2 Indigenous worldviews about courage and fear tend to hold that once one moves from fear to the courage to act, the next step is to fearlessly engage fully with a trust that you are doing your best and whatever happens can be accepted. See Dr. R. Michael Fisher' text (2018) *Fearless Engagement of Four Arrows: The True Story of an Indigenous-Based Social Transformer.* Peter Lang.
3 Remember that if stress or fear can cause an emergency victim to go into spontaneous hypnosis, the same is true for the rescuer. However, the rescuer aware of the power of words while in this state, can quickly put oneself into a light trance, produce a practice directive and believe in the image it produces, and then proceed with full consciousness in the rescue mission.
4 Jacobson, E. (1938). *Progressive Relaxation.* 2nd edition. University of Chicago Press.

3 Rapport

This chapter's primary goal is to teach strategies that will develop trust between the patient and the first responder. Rapport refers to what happens with rescuer and victim are in synch. When this happens, a mutual exchange of verbal and nonverbal communication facilitates a positive relationship that enhances the potential of hypnotic communication. Rapport supports the patient's sense of positive outcomes and thus a willingness to consider whatever the first responder offers. It decreases physical tension and the defensive posture that increases debilitating stress. It opens pathways that can mobilize natural healing capabilities.

Before reviewing some communication strategies and techniques for developing rapport, note that there is one aspect of rapport that cannot be taught. It is an automatic and instant rapport that can sometimes exist between individuals. Such a positive rapport makes it seem like two strangers have had a long and sacred friendship. We mention it here only to let the reader know to look for it as it can be found more often than one might imagine. Another thing to note is that it is difficult or impossible to gain positive rapport when the patient is intoxicated with alcohol or has taken certain drugs. This does not mean you should not try as sometimes such a person will respond extremely well to your words. However, getting such a person's attention can be challenging.

Guidelines for Establishing Rapport

Your first opportunity to establish a positive rapport with a patient is when you arrive at the scene and make initial contact. Rather than starting medical treatment without saying anything (as is often done) take a moment to introduce yourself. If you can obtain the person's name from someone on the scene, do so, but only if the patient cannot speak. If the patient hears you ask someone else, they may feel more of a sense of helplessness than need be, and developing interpersonal rapport with them may be more difficult. Ideally, it is best to get their name by introducing yourself and then asking if the person can tell you what they liked to be called by.

DOI: 10.4324/9781003430261-5

Since the initial contact is at the peak of a first responder's anxiety level, remember to take a moment to gather confidence. Having a plan of action before speaking to or touching the patient will help with this. Then, before beginning extrication or medical treatment, explain who you are and what you aim to do. Give evidence of your respect for the person as someone who will be participating at some level in their survival and healing. If the patient is about your age or younger, use the first name. If the patient is a senior, it may be more respectful to refer to them as Mr. or Mrs. The following examples will give you an idea of how to construct an effective introduction. Modify one of these to suit your own style of communication.

Sample Introductions

- Hello, John. I'm Don. I'm an EMT with the County fire department, and I'm here to help you. I'm going to take care of you, Is that OK? We'll have you out of here soon and you will be on the mend before you know it.
- Mary, I know you're uncomfortable, but the worst is over now, even though it may not seem that way to you. I'm an EMT, and we're here to get you through this. Are you with me on this?
- Bill, my name is Robert Simon, and I can help you, but I want you to help me as best you can. Will you do that? (Say "Good" to any positive acknowledgment or gesture).
- Mr. Jones, I'm James Sheffield and have been a paramedic for over 20 years. I want you to listen carefully to my words now. Can you hear me?

Notice that, in all four examples, several objectives were met. First, each patient was addressed with their own name. This provides recognition and familiarity. Second, each patient was asked a question. This gives a sense of control to the patient at the outset. Third, you have introduced yourself as someone who can help. Fourth, a sense that the future is hopeful is suggested.

If there is no one to tell you the patient's name, then ask it directly, regardless of how severe the injury or illness. If the patient cannot or will not answer you, tell them that that's quite all right, then continue treating the patient and talking to them.

Introduction to a Conscious Patient Whose Name Is Unknown

"Hello, I'm Jim Reeves. I'm a paramedic. Can you tell me your first name? [Patient answers with name.] Good, Bill, we're going to check you over now so we know can determine exactly what injuries you have." In giving you their name, the patient begins to regain a little sense of control. In hearing the name called back, a sense of familiarity and comfort is had.

Introduction to an Unconscious Patient Who Is Breathing

"Hello, Richard I'm David and my partner is Dorothy. We're both Emergency Medical Technicians and we're here to help you. Go ahead and leave your eyes closed for a while longer while we take your blood pressure."

Introduction to an Unconscious Patient Who Is Not Breathing

"Hello, Jean. My name is Josephine and I'm a paramedic. I'm here to help you. I'm going to lift your jaw and tilt your head back to make it easier for you to breathe in this oxygen through the mask you will feel us placing over your mouth." Remember that, *even if the patient is unconscious, it is very important to tell the patient what you are going to do before you do it.* Unconscious patients can, at some level, hear all the words that are spoken in their presence. (More will be discussed about this in Chapter 12, "Cardiovascular Emergencies")

Introducing Humor to Gain Rapport

It can often be helpful to inject some degree of humor into the situation. For examples:

- "Mr. Bell, I know you have better things to be doing on a Saturday night, but here we are and you will at least have an exciting story to tell your friends."
- "Well, Mary, I'm going to cut the sleeve so I can bandage your arm. I hope it is not your favorite shirt!" or "I'll bet you can think of something you'd rather be doing than this."

Of course, a great deal of tact and sensitivity must be used when being humorous at the emergency scene. If you are sincere and caring, however, any effort at humor will usually be helpful. If there is no positive response to your humor, ask the patient "Have you been under any emotional stress prior to the accident?" In many instances, an injury or an accident causes a person to focus on other negative stresses in their life until these cannot be separated from the accident. When you ask this question, the patient has the opportunity to make the separation and thus get on with the process of survival.

The famous physician and hypnotherapist, Dr. David Cheek, once asked this question to a patient brought into the emergency room when he was on duty. The patient was a 42-year-old unmarried woman who had been found unconscious on her living room floor in a pool of blood. When she arrived at the hospital, she appeared to be unconscious, and her skin was cold and mottled in appearance. Her respiration was shallow and rapid; her pulse rate was 140. Dr. Cheek leaned over to her and asked, "Have you been under any emotional stress lately?" This was the first remark anyone had said to her. She opened her eyes and answered,

"Oh, I'm so ashamed. I've been going with my friend now for two years, and I had intercourse with him last night." Dr. Cheek laughed and said, "For goodness sake, why did you wait so long?" At this point, color returned to the woman's cheeks, she smiled and asked Dr. Cheek not to tell her roommate, and her pulse dropped to 100.

Showing Authentic Respect

Respect is a two-way street. If you show respect for patients, they will return the feeling twofold and are likely to do what you say. Sometimes, overworked first responders may show an attitude that sees just another victim. Or sometimes an over-authoritarian approach may be how a seasoned medic deals with emergencies. Although sometimes this may be needed, as we show later, it is usually preferable to treat patients with great respect. This includes sincere attention to their sense of embarrassment, their intelligence, their concerns, and their potential ability to cope, etc. The original desire to help others that brings people into emergency medical service (EMS) can become calloused after many calls. Duty is not the same as sincerity. The most proficient medical treatment without the additional power of effective communication falls short of what should be accomplished for the patient.

This also means respect for the patient's ability to communicate. The patient should not be the last one to have input about their medical problem. When possible, simply asking the patient to describe the problem will build rapport. Similarly, letting the patient tell you what position they are most comfortable in, or asking what they need will help develop a sense of mutual respect. Using the same language as the patient also tends to promote trust if it is done without mockery. If you talk to a construction worker the same way you talk to a college professor or vice versa, you will not achieve optimal rapport. Trust is also threatened if you use baby talk with the elderly or if you are less than truthful.

Showing respect for someone's rights, privileges, and abilities is not the same as a sincere concern for their welfare, but respect and concern for the person's well-being both serve to help you gain a positive rapport. If an emergency patient is convinced that your intentions are totally aimed at their well-being, the trust required for effective communication becomes more likely.

Having such concern for a patient who is a stranger may not be automatic for a first responder, professional, or otherwise. In some situations, the emergency patient may even appear disgusting or unworthy. They may be responsible for having hurt others. If a rescuer has any negative feelings toward the patient, it is unlikely a positive rapport allowing for using emergency hypnosis will emerge. Rescuers should not go through the motions of emergency care without really caring. Finally, if the patient is a loved one or a personal friend, it is important for the rescuer not to show overconcern for their welfare. This could be misinterpreted as worry and could diminish positive rapport to a point where directives are disregarded.

Talking in the Patient's Language

If it can be done naturally, without obvious effort or mockery, talking to a person in their own language facilitates trust. This might include speaking a foreign language when necessary but refers primarily to the style of conversation. Knowing the lingo of different population groups can also be an asset. Talking about subjects that the medic can assume would be of interest to the victim can also build rapport. If you listen carefully to what a patient is saying and how they are saying it, you can learn much about them and use it. For example, if you find the person conveys a sense of courage, talk to them frankly and indirectly acknowledge it. If someone conveys a sense of humor, do your best to offer it back.

Often a style of communication can be determined by observing the clothing of a patient. For example, if a woman is wearing unique, handmade jewelry, she has told you that she is unique and creative. In this case, it would be easier for you to gain rapport by acknowledging this in your communication. For example, you might say to such a person, "What I'm going to ask you may seem a little unusual, but I want you to hold the IV while I check out your leg." Asking them to do anything offbeat that would not be harmful will help you speak their language.

Very simple phrases are often sufficient to put you on a patient's language level. For example, to an army general you might say, "This is the routine thing to do;" to a high school freshman, "Hang loose while I do this;" to a well-groomed in a business suit, "The most efficient thing we can do now is this."

Talking in the patient's language might also mean being in agreement with them. For example, if a patient tells you that they do not trust people in uniform, you might reply, "Sometimes people in uniform can be difficult to get along with, but of course, that isn't always true. In spite of my uniform, I want you to know that I am here to help you" By initially tending to agree with the patient, and then gradually modifying their defenses, you can begin to build on the rapport you gained with the agreement.

Maintain a Proper Balance of Power

Such interplay with patient defenses might be thought of as a balancing of power between victim and rescuer. This is why quickly building rapport is a delicate matter at the emergency scene. When partners are working together, one might focus on rapport building while the other begins physical treatment interventions. When one is alone, building rapport cannot take time away from needed interventions, like stopping bleeding or giving oxygen, but a few proper words while doing these rapport-building things can influence the outcome. A patient monitors their trust carefully. If the "hidden observer" in the patient's mind perceives a threat, rapport is quickly lost. Maintaining a proper balance of power is one way to keep this hidden observer content.

Balance of power relates to the degree of control that is shared between the patient and the rescuer. This is different in every case. Some patients will need more control, some will need less. Furthermore, the degree of power may fluctuate back and forth during a single case.

Determining the balance of power is an experimental process. It is usually best to begin by offering the patient the majority of control and then gradually usurping it as necessary. For example, you might ask the patient to hold an ice pack on an injury, hence acknowledging their power. If, however, the patient does not respond positively to this, the balance of power should shift more to you. If you feel the patient has a high degree of control in a situation, you might ask them to handle pain by saying, "You seem to be handling yourself well; can you stay just as relaxed as you are right now while I take your blood pressure?"

If, on the other hand, the patient does not seem to be in much control, it would be preferable to say, "I know you are uncomfortable, but I want you to listen to me carefully. We are going to do everything we can to help make you more comfortable." In this latter situation, the power shift to the rescuer would be a more effective way to help with the patient's pain. Some degree of power should always be given to the patient, regardless of how much they are willing to take.

An easy way to ensure that this is being done is to *always tell the patient what you are going to do before you do it.* For example, if you are about to put on a blood pressure cuff, you must first say, "I'm going to go ahead and put the blood pressure cuff on your arm so we can get a reading. There you go now I'm going to put some air in it, and you'll notice it becoming more snug."

Occasionally, you will find that a "one-down" position of power will build more rapport than a "one-up" position. An emergency patient is already feeling out of control of their environment and may not need further insult as a result of being treated as an inferior being. If you reveal your own weakness, they may feel less threatened. For example, "Bear with me, if you would. I'm a little slow when it comes to getting a good medical history. I want to make sure to ask all the right questions." This kind of exchange can help not only to iron out any potential power struggle but also to establish a first-name basis between you both.

Make Realistic Statements

Although we discuss this as relates to hypnotic directives in a later chapter, being realistic is important when building rapport as well. When you lose credibility in the eyes of the patient, you lose trust. It is therefore important to make statements that are sufficiently realistic. An example of an unrealistic sentence might be, "There's nothing to worry about," when told to a patient who is uninsured and who just crashed an expensive car into a parked school bus. Although seemingly improbable directives will ultimately be effective at this stage of communication, care must be taken to keep sentences realistic.

This rule is especially critical when dealing with children. For instance, if you were to tell a child that their cut didn't look too bad and that it couldn't hurt too much, you might instantly lose rapport and have difficulty both in patient management and treatment outcome. A more appropriate sentence would be, "Wow, look at that cut—I'll bet that hurts." With this approach, the child would acknowledge that you know what you are doing because you indeed understand how they feel. Then you can begin to change the child's feelings.

Use Feedback Strategy to Gain Rapport

A good communication tool is to be a keen observer. A successful trial lawyer or salesperson, for example, is able to note the needs and concerns of their audience. By addressing such concerns before the listener consciously conveys the information, the speaker presents oneself as someone with special insight— someone who should be trusted. Professional con artists have mastered the feedback strategy to such a degree that, within a very short time, they can cause their targets to entrust them with their life savings.

By being observant of your patient, you can also demonstrate this rapport-building "special insight." Here are just a few examples of feedback strategies.

Situation: The rescuer arrives at a traffic accident, to find a seriously injured twenty-four year old female lying in the street. She is conscious and extremely frightened. Within five minutes the rescuer has completed primary and secondary surveys and all possible field treatments. The patient appears less frightened, and her pulse has lowered. Then the sounds of ambulance and police sirens appear as they approach the scene from about a half mile out. The rescuer's observations of the patient signal that the sirens will trigger increased anxiety, so the rescuer says, "Well, here comes some more help. I know the sirens sound frightening, but they do keep us from getting stuck in traffic."

Having addressed her concern, seemingly before she herself consciously displayed it, the rescuer will have increased rapport while at the same time reducing her anxiety.

Situation: A forty-two-year-old male has suffered burns from an oil tank explosion, and the rescuer has placed an oxygen mask on his face and is administering oxygen. While the rescuer is adjusting the liter flow, he notices the patient start to bring his hand up to the mask and slightly turn his head. The rescuer realizes that the man is about to be bothered by the confining structure on his face. Before the patient's anxiety builds and he tries to remove the mask, the rescuer says, "You might be a little bothered by the mask. Most people are at first. But if you just concentrate on that nice, fresh, relaxing flow of oxygen, you will notice how much more comfortable it can become."

With this sentence, the rescuer will have gained sufficient rapport with the patient to immediately follow with a directive such as "But if you just concentrate on...." As the patient actually becomes comfortable with the mask, he further acknowledges the rescuer's "special insight."

Another way to successfully use the feedback strategy is to simply repeat what the patient has told you afterward. The patient may or may not remember that they gave you the information. In either case, trust in you will be increased when the patient hears you state what they believe to be true. Your statement can be made to another care provider or can be fed back to the patient. The statements can include the patient's stated symptoms, complaints, concerns, desires, and so on. They can also relate to the observation of the patient. For example, if the patient swallows, you might say, "You might notice how soothing it feels to swallow."

Congratulate Patient on Positive Responses

When you commend a patient for following your directions, you enhance rapport with that person. We are accustomed to bonding, with people who congratulate us, whether they have been teachers, parents, coaches, or friends. Do not be overly patronizing with your praise, unless talking to a small child. Simply saying, "That's good," will usually be sufficient. For example, if you ask the patient to take a deep breath and they do, simply say, "Good." When using this approach to specifically develop rapport, be sure to give some directives that you know the patient can and will follow.

Join in with Patient, Then Reframe

Another strategy for assuring positive rapport with a patient is to initially "join in" with that person in their complaint. This could mean an agreement or even a mimicking or sharing of the presenting signs or symptoms. Joining in works especially well with a patient who would be likely to turn off to a rescuer who attempted to directly stop or change their destructive behavior. In most cases, such patients will be highly emotional. This strategy is also very effective with asthma attacks and hyperventilation, or panic attacks.

To join in with a patient in respiratory distress, begin mimicking the patient breathing rate and rhythm while saying, "I know ... how difficult ... it is ... for you to get an easy ... full breath ...." (For an asthma patient this can be done while preparing to administer oxygen.)

At this point, while your breathing rate is in rhythm with the patient's, gradually begin to slow down the rate and watch how the patient will now start to follow *your* lead. As you do so, say, "But notice how much ... easier ... it is becoming to take a nice, easy, full, relaxing breath." When the patient begins to breathe normally, congratulate them by saying, "That's good."

First responders often need to calm an emotionally out-of-control relative. Joining-in strategies can be very helpful in such situations as well. Simply acknowledging the distraught person's feelings can have a noticeable calming effect. Thus, instead of saying, "It's okay. (the patient) is going to be fine. Just calm down," say something like: "I can imagine how frightened you are for (the patient), but we're going to take good care of them." This approach tends to put you in rapport with the concerned by-stander and makes the person an ally rather than someone who might upset the patient.

Situation: Two fire-fighters receive a call to respond to a house where a child was "mauled by sled-dogs." At the scene a 6 year-old female child was screaming convulsively. Her clothing was torn and she was bleeding super-ficially on her head, face, arms, and legs. Her parents and several neighbors said "there are no deep cuts that they could find" and explained she had entered a pen where three sled dogs were confined and they "played rough" with her. They were trying to calm her down by saying she was not hurt badly. Captain Frank kneeled down in front of the child and said "Oh my! Look at all that blood! You must be scared to see all this blood coming out of you!

Instantly the child reduced the intensity of her crying and it was obvious that Captain Frank had achieved a positive rapport. He then said, "Wow, look how that beautiful red blood is helping me clean the dirt of this place" as he was using a 4x4 to clean the wound. "Can you make it bleed just a little more and then stop it for me?" The little girl now had all but ceased her crying and nod-ded her head. The bleeding stopped. The captain then gave her a 4x4 and had her participate in finding other scratches and small punctures, etc.

Divert Attention from Injuries

Whenever an action or statement of the rescuer actually increases the comfort of the patient, rapport is enhanced. Diversion is a relatively easy way to accomplish this. When the patient's attention can be distracted from their problem or pain, there is an actual decrease in the discomfort until their attention again focuses on the problem. When the diversion is a direct result of listening to the rescuer, the patient will associate the temporary relief with the rescuer's words, and rapport is developed. A variety of questions and directions can be used to get the patient to direct attention to something apart from their chief complaint. Asking the person's age, having them pay attention to the blood pressure cuff, or involving the patient in the treatment of a minor complaint— all can serve the purpose.

Another way to achieve diversion is with the secondary survey. Ask the patient to tell you the degree of discomfort felt when you press on a part of their body. Then, intentionally begin to press on an area you know are not involved with pain or injury. As the patient's attention focuses on these places and the pressure of your hand, the patient will momentarily forget the main injury. Subconsciously, this relief will be associated with your words, and this will create a positive rapport, or *transference*. The statement, I'll bet you can imagine someplace else you'd rather be right now, followed by the question, asked matter-of-factly, What would you be doing if you could be doing your favorite thing? Can be very effective in diverting the patient's attention away from pain and discomfort. Very often, the patient will allow their imagination to take them to a warm beach in Mexico or to a hammock under the trees. More will be discussed about such imagery when we discuss expectations and directives.

One quick diversion approach to showing a patient your words can be comforting uses a double-bind tactic. When individuals are in spontaneous hypnosis, either-or thinking becomes more intense as a result of a narrowing of attention. A first responder, after assessing whether or not an arm can be safely moved would simply ask the patient, "Would you be more comfortable with your arm at your side, or here resting on your left?" The patient will likely make a choice. When they do, they have diverted their attention from the pain to something that they have been told will reduce it. Going further, you could say, "Good, now allow that comfort to continue as I bandage the wound." (As we show later, this could lead to a directive to stop bleeding, lower blood pressure, etc.)

Obtain a Direct Contract with the Patient

Most salespeople are taught this tact for bringing a client into a more receptive state for a sales pitch:

> Good to meet you, Mrs. Jones. I'm Bill Sales and I'm here to tell you about this vacuum sweeper. If you could have a sweeper that cleaned the house by itself while you are doing something else would you want it?

If the client says yes, there is a good chance they will buy it. (This is why every state has a law that says a person can change their mind within three days of having been sold something by a door-to-door salesperson. The law recognizes spontaneous hypnosis is operating.) To use this tactic with an emergency patient, you might say: "Hello. My name is John. I'm a paramedic, and I'm here to help you. Will you do what I say so I can make you feel better?" If the patient agrees, this may be all that is needed for him to follow subsequent directives designed to influence critical autonomic functions.

Most of the above communication approaches for achieving rapport have been indirect strategies. In some cases, rapport can be obtained with a direct contract at the outset of care. A direct contract is best attempted when the first responder feels very confident and the patient appears to be very receptive. Otherwise, a rejection of the contract may temporarily block rapport. It should be noted, however, that failure to achieve the direct contract initially is not at all a serious setback. The use of indirect strategies will soon put you back on track.

It is recommended that you study the preceding rapport strategies so that they can be used spontaneously throughout any emergency rescue or patient treatment. When positive rapport is easily achieved with one technique, the use of the others will help maintain it.

When a particular technique does not work for you, continue trying with it and others until rapport is gained or until the patient is no longer in your care. Even if rapport is not gained until after field treatment has been given and the patient is about to be put in an ambulance, its eventual achievement will allow you to offer a departing directive that could significantly affect future treatment outcome. It should also be noted that rapport with a patient might first be gained by a bystander before you arrive. Someone in the crowd surrounding the emergency scene might yell, "Oh my God, that person is going to die if he isn't moved away from the car!" This may have been said with such conviction, sincerity, and authority as to create rapport sufficient for the patient to believe in the statement. Thus, until you are able to establish rapport, it is helpful to keep people in the crowd from interfering when possible.

Transferring Rapport

If you are a first responder and have gained a positive rapport with the emergency patient, it can be troubling to watch your patient being transferred to the care of others who do not have a good rapport and who make no effort to acquire it. To help prevent this from happening, you can transfer your rapport to the next tier of support. The EMS tier of support is as follows:

- First responder (citizen, fire department, etc.)
  - Paramedic
    - Emergency room physician or nurse.

There are essentially two parts to the transfer. The first is a statement to the patient that gives your personal endorsement to the next EMS provider. "Mr. Jones (the patient's name), Bill is an experienced paramedic who works for the city. He will build take over now and build on the care I have begun with you. He's going to check you over and might even ask some of the same questions I did. You're in good hands with him."

The second part in the transfer requires that you inform the next provider that you have gained a positive rapport with the patient and that the patient has been responding positively to your directives. You can make this statement in the presence of the patient if you choose. If the patient hears what you are saying, it can serve to reinforce the statement. So, for example: "Bill, Mr. Jones is complaining of discomfort in his lower right abdomen. I've written down his vitals and response levels for you. He is doing very well and will continue to do so under your care."

In many instances, especially if you have been with the patient for a long time before assistance arrives, you may have given the patient a particular directive that is working very effectively. For example, "Whenever you take a deep breath, your discomfort will lessen." Be sure to share this directive with the next medical provider so they can repeat or reinforce the directive when needed.

True or False

1 To maintain rapport with a patient, it is best to always present a dominant, "one-up" position.
2 Joining in" is not an effective strategy for calming a hysterical person.
3 Asking a patient if they will follow your instructions is one way to achieve rapport.
4 Rapport with the second-in responder will occur automatically if the patient has a rapport with the first-in responder.

Exercise

Write an introductory script you would feel comfortable using in a medical emergency situation. Practice it out loud until it feels natural.

4   Expectation

After positive rapport is established, it is time to give the patient a positive expectation for the immediate future. This chapter presents strategies for creating such expectations that ultimately set the stage for the acceptance of images that could influence the autonomic functions of the body. The following communication strategies can be used to move a patient toward accepting beneficial suggestions that may initially be too unbelievable to accept. Note that one or more of these strategies may be used effectively in less than a minute and will not significantly delay your giving the desired directive.

Use Minor Successes to Achieve Major Ones

A basic principle of motivation is that success breeds success. When we are able to achieve one objective, we are more likely to attempt another. It is therefore wise to start out with relatively easy goals and to work up to more difficult ones. Similarly, when patients act upon suggestions, they become less likely to oppose future ones. Each time a patient successfully follows a directive, expectation is built up for implementing the next one. Therefore, if time permits, it is best to start with easier ones and to work up to more dramatic ones. Easy directives include such things as asking a patient to tell you her name, to hold something for you, to cough or take a deep breath, and so on. After such directions are followed, be sure to congratulate the patient by saying "Good," or "Thank you," so as to frame the response as a minor success.

Give Assurance of a Hopeful Future

The most important thing you can do to build expectations is to give assurance that the patient's future is hopeful. This can be accomplished with both direct statements and indirect statements.

DOI: 10.4324/9781003430261-6

Direct Assurances

With direct assurances, care must be taken to avoid being unrealistic. Sentences such as "Everything is going to be fine," or "There is nothing to worry about," will not be effective. The following examples of direct assurances are more likely to work:

- The worst is over.
- I'm an EMT and I'm going to help you.
- You're going to be OK.
- Things are being made ready for you at the hospital.
- The ambulance is on its way to bring you to the hospital, where the doctors will have you fixed up soon.
- By tomorrow this will just be something for you to talk about.

Indirect Assurances

Indirect assurances, when properly presented, can be the most effective way to reassure the patient. Indirect assurances are statements that imply that the patient will recover from the injury or illness. The following examples can easily be modified to fit the unique circumstances of each incident:

- I've found that many patients are able to_____ after I give them_____. When you get out of the hospital, I'd like for you to stop by the firehouse and say hello.
- It will be helpful when you are better if you try to avoid _____.
- Are you taking a vacation this or next year? Where are you going?
- I have a friend who had the same thing happen to him last year. He still has _____ (describing a minor symptom that would likely result from the injury or illness after initial recovery, only if needed for realism), but otherwise he made a 100 percent recovery.
- When you get well, I'd appreciate it if you would send me the address of the place you bought that (some interesting item owned or worn by the patient that might have value to you).

Thus, any indirect implication that patients will recover and be able to accomplish the requests you present will give them hope and increase their susceptibility to directives that will help them survive and recover.

Make Suggestions Contingent Upon a Physical Occurrence That Will Definitely Happen

With the contingency strategy, the desired objective is described in such a way as to make it seem contingent on something else you are going to do. This is done simply by stating the thing you are going to do or that the patient is going to experience and then suggesting that the patient will also notice some desired objective. The statement should be made in such a way as to matter-of-factly link the two objectives together—that is, to make them contingent upon one an other.

This strategy can be used with a wide variety of medical interventions, from putting on a bandage or elevating the patient's feet to giving medication or administering IVs. In the following examples, a feeling of relaxation is made contingent on the releasing of a blood pressure cuff. (Contingencies work best when there is some obvious association between the two.)

"Now, I'm going to take your blood pressure. As the cuff deflates, notice how much easier your breathing becomes and how relaxed your muscles begin to feel. Good!"

In a sense, the placebo effect is a contingency strategy. Confidently stating what an intervention will do will increase the effectiveness of the intervention. Here are some other examples of contingency strategy.

- This bandage will help stop the bleeding.
- This pill will improve your circulation.
- This position will make you more comfortable.
- If you take a full, deep breath right now, you'll notice that your heart rate will slow down considerably.

Double-Bind Strategy: Offer Two Alternatives, Both Leading to a Desired Objective

If you ask a patient, "Would you be more comfortable with your arm at your side or across your lap?" they are not likely to present a third alternative. When the patient chooses by gesture, silent agreement, or verbal answer, they have accepted a degree of comfort in spite of their predicament. You can increase the focus on this comfort by saying, "Good. Just allow that feeling of comfort to spread through your arm and shoulders." But even without such follow up, the patient's comfort level will have increased enough to build hopeful expectations for more suggestions from you.

The double-bind strategy thus provides the patient with an illusory freedom of choice between two possibilities, neither of which is really acknowledged as desired by them, but may actually be helpful to their welfare. Perhaps the simplest example of this, away from the emergency scene, is when children are reluctant about going to bed. If they are told they must go to bed by 8:00 p.m., they tend to fight against the order. If, however, they are asked whether they want to go to bed at 7:45 p.m. or 8:00 p.m., the majority will select the latter time of their own free will.

A simple double bind is to say, "Let's find out how much comfort this procedure will give you." The tacit implication is that it *will* give the patient comfort; the question is just how much.

Similarly, saying, "You might be surprised to find that you will feel more comfortable," the patient may challenge the statement by not being surprised to find comfort—or indeed to feel surprised at being comfortable.

The combinations of double binds at the emergency scene are limitless (legs up or down, strap tight or loose, blanket on or off), but make sure that both alternatives are appropriate for the medical treatment intended. For example, do not ask a patient who needs to be put in the shock position if she would be more comfortable sitting up or lying down. Although numerous objectives besides comfort can also be used with the double-bind strategy, suggesting that a patient be more comfortable is preferable to phrases such as "less pain," "more oxygen," "less nervous," and so on. More will be discussed about this in Chapter 10, Managing "Pain" ("Discomfort").

If the patient does not answer a double-bind question, this sets up an opening for dropping the suggestion of *your* choice into their subconscious. Research has shown that, when someone is confronted with double-bind choices that are not negative, a disequilibrium momentarily occurs. With emergency patients, this imbalance increases receptivity for a *suggested* choice. Thus, after asking a double-bind question, if the patient hesitates without a reply, simply say, "I think you'll be more comfortable with your hand at your side."

This strategy can also build positive expectations when presented with future alternatives. For example, telling a patient who fears there will be no tomorrow that they will either feel hungry or a little nauseous in the morning, will lend to change their view. (This particular statement would be used only it neither event would be harmful, as the patient will most likely be one or the other if they survive the immediate crisis.) Similarly, double binds can be set up with words like *expectedly* or *unexpectedly* or with phrases like "I don't know *which night* you will sleep the sounder," "if not now," "in a few minutes," and so on.

Guide the Patient's Images Away from the Problem

Positive expectations increase each time an emergency patient perceives a moment of relative comfort. The human mind can be programmed to ignore pain and sources of shock if directed to concern itself with times and places where pain and fear did not exist. If the patient can talk, this technique can sometimes be implemented by simply getting the patient to talk about work, hobbies, or family. If talking does not seem appropriate, or when the patient cannot talk, you can guide their images' elsewhere by asking them to imagine being in a far-off place. A smooth way to use this approach is to simply state, with a little levity, "I'll bet you can imagine someplace you'd rather be than here." Then, while administering medical treatment, ask what her favorite place is. In most cases, the patient will tell you. At that point, matter-of-factly suggest that they go ahead and go to that place in their mind's eye. Tell the patient that they only need to come back when you or another paramedic speak to them. When the patient sees themself, even if briefly, in that place, they will be more calm and reassured. This will in turn increase the patient's positive expectations and inclination to follow your subsequent suggestions or directives. (More detailed description regarding images will be presented in later chapters.)

Sometimes instead of an image that brings the patient's attention away from the painful situation they are in, it may be more beneficial to have the individual focus on the injury, illness or pain in a way that allows for their minds to accept and then modify feelings and outcomes. For example:

> I know how much discomfort you must be feeling in that knee. I want you to focus on it and allow yourself to notice exactly how it feels. Get in touch with what your body is doing to heal it. Begin to allow the discomfortable feeling to change so that you tolerate it better and better as the body's natural mechanisms for healing keep working.

Utilize Ideomotor Response

One way to build the patient's positive expectations is to request for them to answer yes or no to questions by signaling with their fingers. This can be phrased as follows:

> For a few moments, I want you to answer some yes or no questions for me by simply raising your index finger if the answer is yes [point to the patient's index finger and touch it] and the middle finger if it's no [point to and touch the middle finger]. If you don't know the answer or don't want to answer, just raise your thumb. [It's not necessary to touch the thumb.] You don't have to make very much of an effort to raise a finger, just a slight movement is sufficient. In fact, you might be surprised to notice the fingers will seem to answer the questions automatically.

At this point, you should begin to ask the patient appropriate yes or no questions. Depending on the state of treatment, this might include questions pertaining to medical history, the cause of the problem, positions of comfort, and so on. If verbal communication is preferred for these types of questions, you can use ideomotor signals when you begin a summary survey to locate specific areas of discomfort or injury. For example, "When I touch a place on your body, let me know with your fingers if you have discomfort there. Use the yes finger if you do feel discomfort, the no finger if you don't."

The reason ideomotor responses tend to build positive expectations is that they seem extraordinary to the patient, as though the health care provider has tapped a powerful resource. Small motor neurons are activated in the appropriate finger when the patient begins to think of the answer. This results in movement that ranges from a slight twitch to a complete raising of the finger. Polygraphs utilize this effect in a similar way. The paramedic should watch the fingers closely after asking the question. Even if a very slight movement of the finger occurs, congratulate the patient on the response. The patient themself will have noticed the movement, but it will seem to them as though it happened automatically, without effort. (In some cases, the answers themselves may be more truthful than the patient would have wanted to answer. For example, if you asked, "Would you be more comfortable if your mother waits in the next room?" the individual consciously may not have wanted to hurt the mother's feelings and would not have expressed their truest feeling. The ideomotor signal, however, is more likely to react to the basic needs of the person. Since the patient realizes the priority for their own welfare, this also tends to build positive expectations.

Ideomotor signaling obviously also serves the function of two-way communication when it may be difficult for the patient to speak for one reason or another. This could be because of physical injuries, speech impairment, or even crowded conditions with many rescuers talking back and forth. In the latter instance, the ability to communicate with the primary paramedic simply and without effort can be of great comfort to a frightened individual. Of course, this requires that the paramedic give constant attention to the patient and continue to ask questions like, "Are you doing all right?" while rescue efforts are being made.

Another way to utilize ideomotor responses relates to patients who are being tended to while they are sitting upright, if they have the use of their arms and hands. Such patients may be given a pendulum device, such as a 2-inch section of string, or chain with a weighted object on the end. (A paper clip will do.) Ask the patient to hold the end of the string between the finger and thumb with the weighted end hanging down. Their elbow should be resting on the arm of a chair or on their knee. Have the person imagine the object moving back and forth in whatever direction they choose. Although this may seem a bit far out, you can explain that this is simply an easy way for them to increase their comfort while you attend to treatment or wait for the ambulance. When the pendulum begins moving, most patients will be surprised, and the temporary distraction will have served to relieve their symptoms. If they appear surprised, tell them,

> Many people are surprised when they see how they are able to effect a movement of the pendulum by merely visualizing it. It's nothing magic, it just shows how much more control you have over your body than you thought and how much more comfortable you can be.

With this suggestion, positive expectations for the future will have increased. (Note: try the pendulum experiment yourself so you can have confidence in it.)

Eliminate Guilt and Anger

Both guilt and anger are emotions that result in negative expectations if they are not attended to properly. Such emotions are natural and can be beneficial if properly released but are poisonous if left unresolved. This is especially true for emergency patients who often feel guilt or anger in connection with their injury or illness. When we help a patient bring such feelings to a conscious level and then dismiss them, positive expectations are more likely to occur.

A good way to deal with a patient's anger is to change it into *constructive aggression*. Aggression, in its truest sense, simply means forceful action. This does not necessarily imply physical force, but instead the power of energy directed toward an objective. Such energy is natural to humans and should not be restrained. If the injured patient of an automobile accident is angry with the person who ran them off the road and is allowing the anger to build inside, then this emotion will impede their survival and healing mechanism *significantly*. Even if the patient attempts to ventilate the anger by verbal complaints like, "That SOB, he shouldn't have been in my lane!" the emotion remains stuck. Emotions are meant to move us toward constructive action. For example, if we feel fear, we allow it to be an emotion designed to move us toward avoiding it. By encouraging the patient to move into courage and then into a fearless trust, we can reduce the negative potential of fear to create shock are diminish healing. One might tell the victim of a car accident caused by another driver: "I know you're feeling very angry at the person who ran you off the road (joining-in strategy), but let's take that energy and use it to get better now."

A similar approach is necessary for addressing feelings of guilt. Guilt, like anger, impedes the body's optimal healing and supports negative expectations of the future. As anger can be turned into constructive aggression, guilt can be turned into a creative mechanism for personal growth. In fact, guilt is an unnatural form of compassion. If someone feels guilt for having accidentally injured someone else, the paramedic can simply commend the feeling as evidence of natural compassion. When guilt is thus reframed, the patient is able to use the new perspective to learn from and grow with. When emergency patients feel guilty for factors that may have contributed to their situation, they tend to view the pain and suffering as punishment.

By giving an end point to the punishment, pain and suffering can be reduced. The following is an example:

> Are you feeling guilty about having lit that cigarette in front of the gasoline pump? Well, listen, we all make mistakes. Besides, don't you think that what has happened to you up to this point has been sufficient punishment? OK, so go ahead and let that go now, and let's concentrate on getting better.

Use Humor When It Feels Appropriate

Humor can also help dispel anger. Most individuals have enough of a sense of humor, although one's sense of humor varies from one person to the next. A first-responders intuition and style of communication may naturally bring forth the right humor or one can study proven jokes and memories them for use when one feels it might be helpful. If a first responder can manage to get a smile, this can go a long way toward helping the patient. If a patient can manage a laugh, even better. Laughter, like crying, is a catharsis. It releases tension, pain, and stress. When laughing, it is difficult to be afraid. Laughter increases tissue oxygenation, disrupts muscular tension, distracts one from pain, and lower blood pressure (after initially raising it). Laughter also decreases negative expectation and stimulates hope.

Although laughter may seem inappropriate to everyone else involved at the emergency scene, if the rapport between prehospital care provider and patient is high and some aspect of the situation is truly funny or ironic, getting to merely acknowledge the humor in something, if no more than a weak smile, is worth the effort. Of course, be cautious that sufficient tact is used so the patient does not feel that the situation is not being taken seriously.

Propose the Use of "Hypnosis"

Most lay people have acquired definite expectations regarding the word, *hypnosis*. Few understand it for what it really is, but most have a notion of its power. In spite of the many misconceptions that a patient may harbor regarding hypnosis, the mention of it by a prehospital care provider, especially a professional paramedic or physician, may offer special expectations. In fact, if a patient indicates a willingness to use hypnosis to alleviate their symptoms, subsequent directives from the rescuer can be very effective. It is not necessary for the rescuer to induce a hypnotic state, since such a state of consciousness most likely already exists. The proposal can be phrased something like this: "Are you familiar with the use of hypnosis in helping to alleviate symptoms similar to yours? Would you like me to show you how to use it? It can be very effective."

Unless the patient is obviously negative about the suggestion to use hypnosis, the rescuer can continue by using a simple hypnotic "ritual" followed by the desired directive. The ritual need be no more than telling the patient, "OK, I want you to take a deep, relaxing breath. Good. Now, when I count to three, just allow your eyes to close and begin to notice how much more comfortable you are beginning to feel." At this point, a specific directive, phrased according to the guidelines presented in the next chapter, can be given. The expectations associated with the word *hypnosis*, combined with the serious need for help of any kind perceived by the patient, make this an effective strategy in many cases.

Since many of the techniques and strategies for effective communication presented in this book are similar to those used in clinical hypnotherapy, it may be useful to present a brief review of what hypnosis is and what it is not. Hypnosis has been used and well-publicized in the medical profession for almost 200 years. In 1956, the AMA approved it officially. Although it is often thought of as being a tool confined to psychosomatic medicine, it has been extensively used for surgical preparation and recovery. Dentists use hypnosis to control bleeding when operating on hemophiliacs. Many expectant mothers use hypnosis for pain-free labor.

Unfortunately, the mystery behind the power of the mind has encouraged actors, writers, magicians, frauds, and religious leaders to convey the idea of hypnosis inaccurately. This, combined with a skepticism of things we do not understand, has added to the confusion about it.

In formal hypnosis, a client makes an agreement with the hypnotist to willingly suspend certain beliefs and allow ones-self to accept other beliefs for the moment. The language of the hypnotist helps the client's conscious mind to intensely focus so as to cut out other stimuli. This intensity of concentration cuts down barriers and allows the hypnotist's message to enter directly into the unconscious.

One possible concern about actually using the word "hypnosis" at the emergency scene relates to state laws relating to the use of hypnosis. If there is a concern, then it is best to continue the hypnosis language, knowing that you cannot avoid it if the patient is in spontaneous trance, but not to use the word "hypnosis."

Exercises

1 What do minor successes have to do with building expectations?
2 Give an example of a way to indirectly offer a patient a positive expectation.
3 Write a sentence that offers a double-bind to help make a patient feel more comfortable.
4 Why and how do ideomotor responses tend to build hopeful expectations?
5 In your own words, define "hypnosis". And "spontaneous hypnosis."

Part II

5   Directives (An Overview)

The previous chapters have described projecting confidence, building rapport, and creating positive expectations in preparation for giving hypnotic directives. This chapter begins to explain how a first responder can give hypnotic suggestions that can direct the patient's autonomic nervous system functions optimally. Of course, as stated previously, such instructions are always ancillary to standard emergency medical care protocols.

The hypnotic phenomenon has a healing capability because it can overcome limiting beliefs, fears, and/or memories that may otherwise prevent the body from doing what it has the potential to do. A properly worded directive can overcome existing beliefs and allow a patient to control life systems in previously unimagined ways. Hypnotic directives can simply be for calming and reassuring, or they can be more specific. For example, they can be used to reduce blood pressure, decrease inflammation, or stop bleeding. When properly formulated, such directives instantly allow the body to express its full recuperative power.

Directives can be direct, as in, "When I count to three, I want you to go ahead and stop your bleeding here at your wrist while I attempt to enter the car so I can bandage it for you." Or they can be indirect: "While your arm stops bleeding as it is beginning to do now, I'll get a bandage out of the first-aid kit for your cut." Indirect suggestions may work better for the patient who is less frightened and may be somewhat less receptive to a direct suggestion than someone who is more frightened and thus in a deeper state of hypersuggestibility. Remember, it can be presumed that all emergency patients are in an alternative state of consciousness that makes them hypersuggestible. Some, however, will be more deeply focused than others. For those more obviously in spontaneous hypnosis, direct suggestions are very effective. Some obvious signs of this deep state of unconscious activity include:

- Relaxed / smoothe facial muscles
- Eyes wide open, mouth slightly open
- Catalepsy (in extreme cases)
- Lacrimation (tears)

DOI: 10.4324/9781003430261-8

- Fearful reactions to safe communication
- Stunned appearance
- Mechanical movements

Before giving directives, of course, the medic must know what the patient needs to do, and this requires a quick, efficient diagnosis. Is the blood pressure dangerously high? Is inflammation occurring? Is the pain severe? Is sufficient oxygen circulating? Is the patient too cold or too hot? Etc. How accurately the rescuer answers such questions depends upon the level of their first aid-medical skills and their diagnostic ability. If the specific biological, psychological, or physiological needs of the patient are unknown, verbal directives can be more generally oriented toward the patient's getting better.

In any case, orienting the conversation toward a positive healing direction with a confident voice is what is needed in all cases to make positive progress with the patient who is already in a hypnotic state brought on by the emergency. Using general directives that encourage positive images for getting better is most important. The professional first-responders technical knowledge about healing mechanisms, however, allow for more detailed images for the patient to imagine and increases opportunities for developing images. Whatever directives are offered, the wisdom of the patient's body can be nudged into its highest potential for healing, overcoming preconceptions that get in the way. Such preconceptions can produce emotions that activate the amygdala, which triggers the release of stress hormones like cortisol. These hormones raise our heart rate and blood pressure, preparing us for fight or flight even after the time for such a choice has passed.

On the other hand, when a medic can create more positive emotions, they activate the ventral striatum, which lowers stress hormone levels. This helps people to relax and feel calm, which in turn leads toward positive homeostasis. In addition, positive emotions also help to boost our immune system and promote healing. Thus, a first responder, even without yet knowing all the problems going on with the patient, can deliver positive messages. It is this communication from the rescue team that pushes the patient toward optimal healing responses.

Although directives based on knowing exactly what a patient needs may create the optimal hypnotic directives, such knowledge is not necessary. Positive messages move the body toward homeostasis, self-repair, and rejuvenation no matter how they are framed. For example, let's suppose a rescuer directs a patient to dilate vessels around the brain to make a headache patient feel less pain. If the headache is caused by too much dilation it does not matter that you just told the patient technically the wrong thing. The message will auto-correct in most cases, owning to what hypnotists like Ernest Hilgard refer to as a "hidden observer" in the patient's mind that accepts the general intent of the directive but modifies the image to fit the more accurate response.[1] On the other hand, if a negative, pessimistic, or frightening directive is phrased, experience shows that the hidden observer is less efficient in its ability to interpret the optimal response.

Exercises

1 What is the hidden observer?
2 Give examples of direct and indirect suggestions or directives.
3 What are some physical signs that show someone is obviously in spontaneous hypnosis?
4 What benefits come with a positive conversation with the patient versus one that is negative?

Note

1 Hilgard, E. R. (1992). Divided consciousness and dissociation. *Consciousness and Cognition, 1*(1), 16–31.

6   Images

This chapter introduces seven guidelines to help assure that your words evoke positive images in the patient's unconscious mind.

The goal of directives given to the emergency patient is the stimulation of images that quickly program and produce healing processes. Although medically accurate directives based on the first-responder's diagnosis are important in terms of intention, medical accurate details as to the biological functions are not necessary. The general intention is all the patient requires. For example, if the emergency is heat exhaustion, images that relate to cool mists, refreshing cool water, comfortable ocean breezes, or *whatever images the patient associates with becoming cool* can be encouraged. If the emergency involves a lacerated organ, imagery might relate to skillful carpenters entering into the bloodstream, finding the organ, and patching it. This image could be the rescuer's creative idea, or the rescuer may ask the patient to relate what they imagine when thinking of something getting repaired. In the latter case, if the patient answers a carpenter, then the rescuer can build on this image by using a metaphor such as "just as if you were fixing a wooden chair broken, you can imagine the body's processes for beginning to heal your injured arm."

The power images have over our actions and normal mode of thinking is depicted by the following illustration: If a 4-inch plank is set on the ground and you are asked to walk the length of it, you would probably have no problem, assuming you had the physical skill to do so. However, if it is placed between the roofs of two tall buildings and you are asked to walk across it, the *imagined* possibility of falling would have more influence over your balance than even a high monetary incentive to accomplish the task. Even if you tried you would likely fall. It is the creative part of guiding images that the first responder may find the most challenging. This is only because of inhibitions about such childlike communication at the emergency scene. Our culture has tended to discourage, rather than encourage, such imaginative discourse. Fantasy has been relegated to the nonproductive side of our existence. The irony is that most of the billions of brain cells we possess relate not to logical, linear thinking, but to imaginative thinking. This inhibition to describe such imaginary ideas will quickly disappear

DOI: 10.4324/9781003430261-9

as the effectiveness of such communication becomes more and more obvious. The following guidelines, combined with a willingness to express your own natural creative imagination, are all that is necessary to help a patient develop healing images.

Utilize All Five Senses When Developing Imagery

When we think of imagery, we often think only of visual imagery. However, imagery can also involve the senses of touch, taste, hearing, and smell. In fact, when several senses are combined, images tend to be more vivid. For example, a person might be more apt to respond to an image of being relaxed by the ocean if he could feel the warm sand, hear the ocean waves crashing into the shore, smell the seaweed and kelp, taste the salty mist, and see the blue skies and green, frothy ocean.

Make Language Understandable to the Patient

The less left-brain activity required to comprehend directives, the more right brain image-producing activity will be available. It is therefore important to speak clearly, slowly, and in terms the patient can easily understand without having to think about meanings. By avoiding any ambiguity in your language, you will help the patient create images quickly.

For similar reasons, it is also helpful to make use of the patient's language. This means speaking in a person's native language when possible. If a patient is bilingual, it is an advantage to speak in the individual's first language. This is because, during early childhood, this language was associated with much imagination. Also, it was the language that authority figures like mother and father spoke, and it may facilitate rapport. Making use of a patient's language also means using slang or regional or occupational phrasing if the paramedic is familiar with it. When this is done, however, care should be taken to do so without parody or seeming to put the patient down.

Use the Patient's Own Experiences

Imagery works best when it is the patient's images that are used, not the rescuer's. A place that is relaxing to one person is not necessarily going to be relaxing to someone else. For example, a paramedic may ask the patient to imagine lying in the sun on the beach because that is *their* idea of being relaxed. The patient, however, may have had a bad experience in such an environment that was anything but relaxing. It is thus always better to ask the patient what a relaxing place for them would be. Then you can direct them to go there and encourage associated images to form.

The author has asked hundreds of emergency patients to describe a happy, comfortable place with the following wording: "I'll bet you can imagine someplace you'd rather be than here right now." Then, after a few moments of working on the patient, ask, "What place did you imagine when you thought of a place you'd rather be?" Almost without exception, patients in all levels of distress have identified a unique spot.

Be Descriptive

Since the emergency patient is not going to feel much like talking, it is up to you to embellish an image with descriptive details so as to color it and make it potent. The following experiment may illustrate the importance of descriptive adjectives when stimulating imagery. Read it through, then set the book aside and try it.

While resting comfortably in your chair or bed, allow your arm to rest at your side. Now imagine that your arm is raising upwards. Do this for a few moments. Whether it raises or not, note and remember what sensations you were feeling or what you were thinking.

Now, refocus on your arm again and the imagined levitation again, but this time, imagine that a bunch of brightly colored helium balloons—red ones, blue ones, green ones, and many of your favorite colors—are all tied by a string to your wrist. See them uplifting in the clear, blue sky. Believe in the image without thinking. Notice how they rise when a brisk summer breeze blows them. You might also imagine them becoming bigger with each breath you take, causing your hand and arm to lift ever higher. Stay with it sincerely.

Now, compare this second experience with the first. In most instances, the latter image will have been more effective in causing the arm to lift than the first one. The more colorful the description, the more vivid the image. Thus, with a patient of cold exposure, you would not just have that person imagine a warm place, you would have them imagine the following: being in the warm sand, feeling the hot sun rays beating down, or, being wrapped in a cozy, soft blanket in front of a big stone fireplace, with the orange flame reflecting heat all over their body and the aroma of a burning oak filling their nostrils. Tell the patient to imagine hearing the crackling and sparkling of the burning embers and their body becoming warmer and more comfortable.

Use Emotional, Exciting Words

Besides being descriptive, your words should have an emotional, exciting intonation and emphasis. It is not known exactly why this increases the imagery potential, but it is thought that it relates to early childhood imagination experiences. During this time, parents and other adults typically speak to children with a tone of emotional excitement in an effort to encourage positive images. For instance, "What a *big* boy! You lifted that *great big brown box all* by yourself," or "What a *beautiful* picture you have drawn. Just look at the *pretty red* flowers." Apparently, such language during times of stress tends to stimulate latent imagery cells and also tends to encourage increased receptivity to parental-type guidance and assistance.

Thus, instead of saying, "Your heart is beginning to beat more regularly now," say "*All* the fibers of your heart muscle are beginning to work *together* now as a *team, pumping fresh, oxygenated blood* to *all* of the cells in your body." The tone of excitement and emotion in your voice will intensify appropriate images and will also seem to validate them. (If you doubt the power of emotional rhetoric, tune in to a TV evangelist and see how they are able to motivate people to contribute to their organization!)

Use Only Positive Phrasing

One of the most important things to remember when speaking to emergency patients is to phrase your statements in the positive. Words like *not* or *won't* do not form images in the mind; therefore, images are produced by the object of the sentence that uses them. Directives that contain negations should therefore always be rephrased.

Wrong way: You're not dizzy any more.
Right way: You're feeling clear-headed.
Wrong way: In a few moments you won't feel like crying.
Right way: In a few moments you will feel more relieved.
Wrong way: Don't breathe so fast.
Right way: Breathe slower.
Wrong way: You are not going to die.
Right way: You are going to live.

The following example demonstrates this point: Susan, a golfer, wants to hit the ball down the fairway in between two ponds. If she says to herself, Don't hit the ball in the pond, or I will not hit the ball in the pond, what happens? The image-producing quality of the words *pond, hit,* and *ball* overshadows the word *not*. As a result, subtle body messages will tend to hit the ball into the pond as imagined. If, however, the golfer says to herself, I will hit the ball *down* the fairway, she is more likely to do so.

In addition to negative statements, words with negative connotation should be avoided. The most common such word used in communication with emergency patients is *pain*. When a paramedic or a physician asks the patient if they have pain or where the pain is, that act has offered the image of pain to the patient. Since any phrase that uses the word *pain* is still going to nurture the image, it should almost always be replaced with the word *discomfort*.

Wrong: Tell me where you feel pain.
Right: Tell me where you feel the most discomfort.

By using the word *discomfort* instead of *pain*, you are now able to form a directive to reduce the pain without using the word—for example, "Notice how much *more comfortable* you are becoming." A good way to work with pain is to ask the patient to describe his discomfort on a scale of 1–100. Then, using the strategies that have been discussed and the examples in Chapter 10, "Managing Pain," ask the patient to see themself at improving levels.

Remember, if the patient can hear what you are saying, it is important to substitute the word *discomfort* for the word *pain* when reporting the injury to the hospital or to personnel taking over the treatment.

Attach Triggers to Images When Called For

A *trigger* is a symbolic action that reintroduces a helpful image automatically. For example, you might tell a patient that whenever they touch their finger and thumb together, the feeling of comfort will quickly and automatically return. Shrugging the shoulders, smiling, taking a deep breath, blinking the eyes, and so on can serve as a trigger. Triggers give the emergency patient a sense of security and control. When being transported to the hospital and away from your confident directives, a patient can use the trigger whenever needed to keep your directives working if and when other reactions temporarily block them.

> *Situation: A patient with a crushed hand has been treated by the rescuer and is responding well to suggestions for pain management. The ambulance has arrived, and the patient is about to be lifted onto the stretcher. The rescuer speaks to the patient:*

Louis, if later on you need to regain the feeling of relative comfort that you are feeling now, all you need to do is take a deep breath, exhale, and touch your finger and thumb together. As soon as you do, that feeling of comfort will come flooding back automatically. Go ahead and do that now. Take a deep breath, exhale, and touch your finger and thumb together. Notice how much more comfortable that makes you, even now. Good.

True Or False?

1 When developing imagery, only the visual sense should be targeted.
2 A day at the beach would be a relaxing image for everyone.
3 "You are not dizzy now," is a proper directive.
4 A trigger helps a patient bring back a useful image.

7 Believability

Since the patient is aware at both the conscious and unconscious level, directives must appear relatively believable, or they may not work. This chapter presents rules that will help the patient believe sufficiently in the first responder's words by moving beyond previous limits to their imagination.

Relatively Believable Directives

Choosing to create the learning mnemonic, CREDIBLE, hints at the importance of this chapter. A first responder must give directives that are likely to be accepted as doable by the patient. Keep in mind that when in a spontaneous trance and fearful setting, most people will not be thinking with their usual critical mind. A fellow rescuer or medic might not believe that imagining falling snow on a burned hand could do anything, but to a patient who is in a trance much more is possible. Your patient can easily accept the notion you design when following the guidelines presented. If you ask a patient to imagine cool falling snow on their burned skin, the act of speaking in ways that convey absolute certainty-inflammatory responses can indeed be reduced. Images follow beliefs and beliefs are nurtured by a sense of credibility.

Directives Should Be Relatively Accurate

A patient does not have to imagine exactly what biological or physiological processes are supposed to be happening. In hypnosis metaphors generally work well. During medical emergencies, "cognitive processes change, becoming literal and overly sensitive to both direct and covert meanings of communicated messages."[1] If directives are too exaggerated, however, belief in them may be challenged by the patient both at a conscious level and at an unconscious level. For example, if when using the aforementioned clean falling snow imagery to help reduce inflammation the medic added a minute later: "In a minute or so your hand will be completely healed," this could be too unbelievable for the patient.

DOI: 10.4324/9781003430261-10

Incorrect directives that disrupt believability usually result from violating one or more of the following:

1   Be honest and as accurate as possible, *without* validating the patient's concerns and fear. Such honesty help maintain the medic's projection of confidence.
2   Use what medical knowledge you have that is most relevant to what body functions your diagnosis thinks are most important. This does not necessarily mean you must be perfectly detailed with your language. If you are encouraging someone to manifest images that will enhance the immune system, it is not essential that you describe biological processes relating to various cellular activities that are involved. It would be sufficiently accurate to speak of immune cells banding together to rid the body of infection, while other cells relax.
3   Show respect for the patient's intelligence but hold back unnecessary information that could disrupt their focus on relatively believable potentialities related to your words. There is often a delicate line between telling the patient possibly frightening information, such as informing a car crash victim that one of her family members was badly injured.

> *Situation: An automobile accident with multiple casualties has occurred. The rescuer is treating the adult driver who has possible spinal injuries and broken ribs. This patient's young child, age ten, is dead. The rescuer knows this. The injured driver does not.*

Patient: Where's my little boy? How is he? Oh my God, is he all right? Please, someone, tell me!

Rescuer: I know how worried you are about your son. There's a paramedic working with him right now, and he's an excellent paramedic. I know he is taking good care of him. The best thing *you* can do for him is to help me do everything we can for you, too. You can begin by keeping your head still while I put on this brace. While we're doing this, I want you to...

In this delicate situation, the rescuer manages to be accurate and honest without revealing information that could be detrimental to the patient's survival potential.

> *Situation: A right-handed thirty-four-year-old male has maimed his right hand in machinery at work. Future use of the hand is unlikely. The patient appears in control and has looked at his hands.*

Patient [speaks after treatment for pain and bleeding has been administered]: Will I ever be able to use my hand again?

Rescuer: I truthfully don't know. I do know that they can do incredible things with reconstructive surgery and that injuries almost always look much worse than they are. You'll probably be surprised to see how much you can do with that hand after a while.

This illustration shows that the amount of information you reveal to the patient is in part determined by how much the patient already knows. Believability is risked if you contradict what the patient knows for sure. At the same time, however, care must be taken not to validate the patient's negative beliefs. Another way to increase believability is to start with a relatively easy directive and work up to more profound ones. A basic principle in psychology that relates to suggestibility is that suggestions that are acted upon create less opposition to subsequent ones.

Use the Progressive Form of the Present Tense When Phrasing Directives

Although a direct imperative like, "Stop your bleeding *now*," can be effective, directives are more likely to be effective if they are phrased to give the patient more leeway to accept the appropriate images—for example, "Your arm is already beginning to feel numb," or "Notice that your arm is beginning to feel numb." This type of phrasing suggests that the patient should become aware of something that is already happening, but they may not have noticed it yet. With this approach, there is less chance that the victim will resist a directive. There is also less chance that rapport will be lost because something you said did not happen right away. Instead, the patient has time to work up to the image.

Forming directives in the present progressive also helps prevent the patient from trying too hard to comply. Another basic tenet of psychology is the law of reversed effect. This says that the harder you try to do something, the more likely it is that you will fail. A directive like "Lower your body temperature, now," may increase activity in the left brain where a willful determination is initiated. However, unless strong, positive success images also exist, willful determination involved in trying to do something somehow reinforces images that relate to the difficulty or inability to be successful. For instance, the harder you try not to blush, the more likely it is that you will blush, and so on. Present progressive directives seem *to assume* success rather than demand it.

Make Directives Relative to the Patient, Not the Environment

Directives are believable or possible when they relate to potential changes in the patient, rather than those things outside them. This is because, in fact, the patient's images can only influence her own mind–body complex, not external objects, persons, or events.* The following examples illustrate this point:

Wrong way: Notice how much cooler it *is* outside.
Right way: Notice how much cooler *your body* is becoming.
Wrong way: Imagine how quickly the help will come.

Right way: Help is on its way. You might be surprised to see how fast the time
will go by until they arrive.

Wrong way: The ride to the hospital will be quiet and relaxing.

Right way: Notice that all the sounds you hear, including the siren and traffic
noises, will *add* to your experience of comfort and relaxation.

As with most rules, this one has an exception. It is all right to direct an image that
relates to what a medication will do as opposed to how the body will react to the
medication, though a directive could be formed either way. As with the placebo
effect, belief in the external power of the substance triggers internal images.
Ultimately, however, it is the belief in what the drug will do for the body that
can influence its success or failure. (Refer back to the experiment with ipecac in
Chapter 1, "Credibility.")

Exercise

Give five directives for five different emergency situations, using the progressive form of the present tense.

*There are hints of evidence that an individual's images *can* affect external reali-
ties. Theories relating to this have been presented in the arenas of philosophy
and, more recently, in quantum physics. Whether such psychic energy actually
exists is a question that may be someday answered when the disciplines of psychology, philosophy, medicine, neurophysiology, and other physical science join
forces. Until then, we might assume that, at least indirectly, what we imagine can
influence the world outside us. (See Chapter 19, "Saving the Planet.")

Note

1 Karnatovskaia, L.V. et al (November, 2020). Stress and fear. *May Clinic Proceedings*,
   95, 2303. https://www.ncbi.nlm.nih.gov/pmc/articles/PMC7606075/

8   Literal Interpretation

Within the first hour after the medical emergency or trauma, the patient is vulnerable to the statements made by others. This mental state exposes the patient to a hyper-suggestible condition that fully evokes a hypnosis situation. That means the things being said around that patient could have a greater impact than they would otherwise because the patient is already hypnotized. Therefore, during the first hour or so, we propose that a person in a trauma-induced trance may be more likely to interpret statements in a literal manner. This chapter helps clarify how to avoid words that can be interpreted literally in ways that can be harmful.

Literal Interpretations of Language in Hypnosis

Most assertions about hypnosis are controversial, as it remains a phenomenon too complex for scientific certainties. Some studies have shown that people in hypnosis take what is said literally. For example, in normal waking consciousness if someone asks you "Can you tell me your name?" you would probably tell them your name. In trance, you would be more likely, according to some studies, and the authors experience in emergency settings, for a response to be "Yes I can." In other words, the question is literally understood as wanting to know if you *can* say your name. Adam Eason gives another example:

> One lady hypnotized herself to sleep better and used the words with herself "when I get out of bed, I feel awake and ready for the day ahead, full of energy" which sounds harmless and well-intentioned, yet she claimed that she got up in the middle of the night to go to the toilet and the effect of the hypnosis suggestions were that she then felt totally awake and alert and had to go about her business, despite it being 3 AM.[1]

Eason's online article goes on to cite hypnosis scholars and studies who say such literalness is a common feature of hypnosis and others that show it is so only in a relatively small number of individuals. Since none of the studies relate to trauma-induced spontaneous hypnosis, we believe in the studies he points

DOI: 10.4324/9781003430261-11

out that emphasize literal interpretations to be important for first responders to assume.

Another aspect of literalness relates to the power of words themselves. Four Arrows offers an example of this from his sports hypnosis work. One example was a golfer, client who, after learning self-hypnosis, failed to heed the literal problem. At a sand trap he went into a trance during a professional game and gave himself the directive: "I will not hit the ball in the sand trap." Of course, that is where he hit it because the words most likely to form images are "hit," "ball" and "sand trap." The proper directive would have been to say: "I will hit the ball into the fairway."

Thus, to help assure that directives achieve the desired results, the paramedic must remember that their words will be interpreted quite literally by the patient. Images are stimulated by their initial perception of meanings. Analytical brain functions that might otherwise be able to put the word or words into context are not operating during stress.

The following practices offer guidelines that will help assure that directives will take literal interpretation into consideration:

Avoid Phrases with More Than One Meaning

Generally, rescuers can avoid literal misinterpretation by keeping conversation simple and patient-directed. When slang or conversational phrases that could be misinterpreted by the patient are avoided, whether to the patient or between rescuers, the chances of such problems are significantly diminished. The old joke common around fire departments depicts this point well. (It probably actually happened once upon a time!) It goes something like this: "Did you hear about the accident patient who was pinned inside their car? The patient didn't have any injuries but died of a heart attack after hearing the fireman call for the 'Hurst'!"

Firefighters usually get this joke because they use the word *Hurst* to refer to a hydraulic rescue tool also called the "jaws of life," which is used to open crushed-in doors. The tool is manufactured by a company called HURST. Obviously, the subject of the story (the patient) thought that the call for a "hearse" implied death. So, avoid phrases that may have more than one meaning. Putting someone to sleep may mean something quite different to the patient who just put his German Shepherd to sleep than to the anesthetist who was merely referring to a general anesthetic.

It is not too difficult to choose sentences carefully when speaking directly to the patient. It is more difficult to control them when speaking to others. Remember that the patient's entire focus of attention is related to their predicament. As a result, anything that is said before a patient is construed as pertaining to them. If the patient overhears someone saying, "He's not going to make it this year," a statement referring to the paramedic's son's prospects for making the football team, the patient assumes the sentence is about themself. The patient assumes that no one could be talking about football when their life is on the line. Even seemingly innocuous phrases like, "He's out to lunch," could damage the patient. A paramedic may simply be telling their dispatcher that one of the paramedics is on a lunch break. The patient may interpret the phrase to mean their condition is much worse than they imagined. Taking a few moments to think before speaking with this point in mind is an important rule for effective communication with the emergency patient.

Affirm Activity, Not Ability

A second guideline that relates to the patient's literal interpretation of communication is to make sure directives describe *activity*, not *ability*. For example, telling a patient, "Notice that you have the ability to stop your bleeding," is not as effective as saying, "Notice that your bleeding is beginning to stop." If the patient accepts the image of the first directive, they will indeed believe they have the ability to stop bleeding, but the mind will not direct the body to do it.

Similarly, the use of the word *try* should be avoided because of the literal translation. If you direct a patient to try and breathe regularly or to try to be more relaxed, the patient will literally *try*. Only when your directive says, "You are breathing more regularly" (direct) or "You are beginning to breathe more regularly" (present progressive), will the desired objective occur.

Simple biofeedback exercises demonstrate the ineffectiveness of "trying," even with people who are not under stress. When hooked up to biofeedback monitors, participants who are not trained in imagery, self-hypnosis, or relaxation responses increase anxiety profiles when asked to try to relax.

Many people are drawn to the field of emergency medicine because of the joy of going to work every day and experiencing something new and exciting. At some point, the experience level builds to a level where some things become routine that are not normal experiences for everyone. For example, an experienced paramedic may have cared for a large number of patients who are near the end of life or actively dying. These situations are a big deal to everyone, especially the family and the patient. But to the experienced paramedic, it may feel like a routine day at the office. This feeling of routine is something you must fight as a provider because it prevents you from being there in the moment with the patient so you can make use of the hypnotic trance affecting of the hypnotic trance affecting them.

Prior to understanding how hypnosis affects the emergency patient it seemed like the main focus of the ambulance response was to figure out what was going on with the patient and make any necessary interventions. Now that you are learning about the psychological elements that are involved, it is easy to see that the interventions can be more than giving treatments like oxygen and IV medications. Working to communicate in a way that is sensitive to the hypnotic trance they are experiencing requires your full attention throughout the entire patient encounter. This helps protect the patient from phrases that would be taken literally. This same degree of attentiveness is required in monitoring how you project yourself. The next chapter will describe the role of enthusiasm in how you communicate during patient encounters.

Exercise

Give three examples of words and phrases that could have more than one meaning.

Note

1 Eason, A. (2011). Do people really respond literally to suggestions in hypnosis? https://www.adam-eason.com/do-people-really-respond-literally-to-suggestions-in-hypnosis/

9 Enthusiasm

The last letter of our CREDIBLE mnemonic is a reminder of the importance of enthusiasm when you are involved in assisting an emergency patient. This chapter describes how the right amount of enthusiasm, not too much nor too little, can be a significant factor in patient communication.

The Role of Enthusiasm in Patient Communication

The right amount of enthusiasm underlies success in projecting confidence, gaining rapport, building positive expectations, and giving successful directives. If the strategies that have been discussed are not working for you, increase or decrease your enthusiasm and note the difference.

What exactly is enthusiasm, how do you get it, and how can it benefit communication with the emergency patient? The word itself comes from the Greek word *enthousiasmos* meaning "inspired." Webster defines it as "ardent interest." Synonyms include the following: *vigor, energy, animation, drive, esprit de corps, potency, spirit, vitality, and devotion.*

Note that all of these qualities enhance the characteristics of leadership. They are things that make a patient want to follow your directives with equal enthusiasm. If you are without enthusiasm at the emergency scene and an enthusiastic bystander is talking nearby, the *patient may focus on the bystander's words and not yours.* Since the bystander has not learned the principles of effective communication, they may very well say something that could significantly hinder the recovery of the patient.

Your level of enthusiasm, especially while at an emergency scene, is determined by your emotional reactions to people and events. These reactions, no matter how internalized they may seem to you, emit energies that are picked up by the emergency patient. Any reaction that negates your energy, your devotion, your esprit de corps, your inspiration, or your potency robs you of enthusiasm.

To get an idea of how a statement without enthusiasm compares to different levels of enthusiasm. For example, try the phrase: "The worst is over now,

DOI: 10.4324/9781003430261-12

and things are being made ready for you at the hospital." Start without any conviction, emphasis, sincerity or sense of importance. Just say it as though you were tired, bored, and/or unconcerned. Notice how it would sound to a patient.

Next, repeat the sentence, this time with what you feel is just the right amount of enthusiasm. Be convincing and caring. Be alive and put your own personality and style into it. Now, imagine how the patient would respond. Practice different levels, noting how too much can be as bad as too little.

Enthusiasm and Self-awareness

Practicing how to communicate does not mean you are learning to fake enthusiasm. It is about self-awareness and it relates to authentic degrees of enthusiasm that you act out with real situations in mind. Enthusiasm also relates to one's style and personality. Using the following psychological traits, score yourself on how much or how little of each trait you now possess. Think of these in relation to how you behave at the emergency scene.

Desire	1	2	3	4	5
Assertiveness	1	2	3	4	5
Sensitivity	1	2	3	4	5
Tension Control	1	2	3	4	5
Confidence	1	2	3	4	5
Personal Accountability	1	2	3	4	5
Self-Discipline	1	2	3	4	5

Take the trait of assertiveness, for example. Assertiveness is the feeling that you can affect the treatment outcome of a patient. Give yourself a low score if you are easily intimidated by a patient, a situation, or other rescuers. Give yourself a high score if you are not. Also, take a low score if you are too assertive to the point of being insensitive. Over-assertiveness can be a greater problem than under-assertiveness because it manifests as insensitivity. (Picture the paramedic who arrives at the scene, ignores the first responders, and goes right to the patient without asking questions, then proceeds to cut the patient's clothes off while giving orders to everyone in an aggressive tone.) If your score is near the middle, your emotional inactions to things that relate to your assertiveness are probably not going to affect your enthusiasm negatively.

Emotions and Enthusiasm

It is important to note your and the patient's emotions as a way to measure your level of enthusiasm. Emotions such as fear, anger, jealousy, anxiety, worry, insecurity, and embarrassment all can dictate the right amount of enthusiasm for different directives. Of course, a task for the rescuer is controlling emotions. When employing one's own enthusiasm for the sake of a patient, such self-control is essential for addressing the emotions of the patient.

Stay in the Present Moment

Whether or not you go to the trouble to work through the previous exercises, your level of enthusiasm will improve if you understand the connection between enthusiasm and serenity. This relationship is best described by the anonymous authored serenity prayer:

"God, grant me the serenity to accept the things I cannot change, The courage to change the things I can, And the wisdom to know the difference."

In a sense, enthusiasm exists in its most perfect form when one is able to accomplish all three of these objectives. Furthermore, this is best accomplished if you can learn to concentrate fully on being in the present moment. This is true because the only way to be in the present is when you *instantly accept emotionally whatever happens at the emergency scene*. This point is well illustrated by the Zen story of a monk who was being chased by two tigers. He came to the edge of a cliff. He looked back—the tigers were almost upon him. Noticing a vine leading over the cliff, he quickly crawled over the edge and began to let himself down by the vine. Then, as he checked below, he saw two tigers waiting for him at the bottom of the cliff. He looked up and observed that two mice were gnawing away at the vine. Just then, he saw a beautiful strawberry within arm's reach. He picked it and enjoyed the best-tasting strawberry in his whole life!

Notice that the monk fully responded to the physical danger in the most intelligent way. His emotional reactions did not relate to his past or future fears or concerns. By being in the present, the emotion that emerged was enthusiasm. This is what the emergency patient most requires.

If being in the present nurtures enthusiasm in the rescuer, would being in the present also be beneficial for the patient? Some evidence indicates the answer is yes. Although patients need positive expectations for a hopeful future to *replace* negative expectations, once this is achieved, the individuals do better when their thoughts remain in the now.

Wrong: Go ahead and think about how nice it will be to be with your family later, and notice how much better you will feel.

Right (after negative worries for the future have been canceled): Notice what is going on around you. Let all the sounds become part of your experience of comfort.

One of the most effective approaches to building appropriate enthusiasm, for both rescuer and patient, is to reframe or redefine problems as being challenges.

It is difficult to face problems with enthusiasm, but challenges can always be met enthusiastically.

Wrong: I know this is a terrible problem for you, but we are doing our best to help you with it.
Right: This may be one of the greatest challenges you will ever have to face, and it offers a great opportunity for you to show how well your inner resources can respond.

Put yourself in the patient's place and hear both statements. Which one is most likely to promote life-embracing enthusiasm?

True or False?

1 Directives should stimulate only images that involve visual sensations.
2 The following directive would be appropriate: "In a few moments, you won't feel any pain."
3 If one directive is followed, a second directive is less likely to be successful.
4 The future tense should always be used when phrasing directives.
5 The following directive would be appropriate: "You now have the ability to lower your blood pressure."

Exercise

Imagine yourself at an emergency scene and see an event that relates to a personality trait and to an emotion. After you have done this, substitute a more appropriate emotional response and mentally rehearse it with the same emergency scene. With practice, the reactive emotion will become reprogrammed and your self-rating for the trait will change.

10 Managing "Pain" ("Discomfort")

This chapter discusses appropriate language to use with people complaining of severe pain. Note that although we use the word "pain" in this chapter for instruction purposes, at the scene of an emergency it is best to use the word "discomfort." This is important because people generally accept various levels of discomfort, but the word "pain" tends to be interpreted with more trepidation and is more difficult for a patient to modify or reduce. Therefore, avoid the word "pain" altogether, especially when communicating examples that have a goal to promote healing.

Pain Management

The emergency patient's tolerance for pain is influenced by a class of biochemicals called endorphins. These are substances very similar to morphine but are produced by the brain. Endorphins block pain by filling specific neuron receptors so that other chemicals that carry pain messages cannot enter. Exactly what causes the production of endorphins and what regulates the amount of these endorphins is not fully understood. What is known is that emotions, attitudes, thoughts, and external verbal and nonverbal communication can significantly influence the production of endorphins. Research shows that pain comes from "an integrated networks that involve activity at multiple eortical and subcortical sites" that can be influenced by hypnosis.[1]

Since methods of pain control are relatively easy to measure experimentally, numerous studies have been done in this area. In most cases, the opiate-like substances produced by the brain proved to be more potent than the administration of pain-killing drugs. This was confirmed back in 1977 when a National Institute of Health study, published in Volume 296 of the *Annals of the New York Academy of Sciences* compared hypnosis, acupuncture, morphine, valium, aspirin, and placebos in the management of experimentally induced pain. Tolerance of pain was measured by a timed exposure to an ice-cold surface and ischemic pain resulting from a blood pressure cuff set at 300 mmHg. With both types of pain, the most significant protection was afforded by the hypnotic suggestion of

DOI: 10.4324/9781003430261-13

analgesia. (The second most effective was 10 milligrams I.M. of morphine per 70 kilograms body weight.). A more recent study (2020) in Medscape showed hypnosis reduced reliance on morphine.[2]

Thus, the experience of pain appears to be largely subjective. You may recall emergency patients with relatively minor injuries expressing extreme pain and others with more severe injuries expressing little. You may also remember the emergency patient who did not complain of pain until you started talking. In these instances, the painful *sensation* of the injury did not become the painful experience of suffering until communication triggered an inappropriate subjective thought about the injury.

If pain is not being expressed by the patient on a conscious level, either verbally or nonverbally (indicated by grimacing, muscular tension, etc.), then there the medic should assume there is no pain experienced. Do not create a pain experience with inferences that pain must exist. The easiest way to do this is to simply avoid using the word *pain* at all in your communication. If you need to ask the patient questions about their pain during the assessment, phrase your sentences more in line with the following example.

> *Situation: The rescuer arrives at the scene of an emergency involving a forty three-year-old male who has fallen from a 14-foot ladder. He is on his back—alert and conscious—and is exhibiting no signs of pain. After checking for bleeding, and while putting on a C-collar, the rescuer begins his secondary survey to determine where the patient is injured.*

Wrong: Mr. Bloom, before we can help you we need to know where you are *hurting* or where you are feeling the most *pain.*

Right: Mr. Bloom, so we can know where to begin, it would help us if you could describe exactly what place on your body needs attention. (Note there is no reference to the "pain" per se.)

Similarly, during the secondary survey with a patient who is not expressing pain, avoid the use of the words "hurt" and "pain," which are likely to start subjective responses that will increase the pain experience. Instead, use the word "discomfort."

Wrong: Tell me if I touch a place where you feel pain.

Wrong: Tell me if I find a place that hurts.

Right: Tell me if I touch a spot where there is some discomfort.

If you are called to an emergency where the person is in obvious pain, there are a variety of directives you may choose from to alleviate the patient's perception of pain, thereby encouraging the production of endorphins. One or more of the following techniques can be used without interrupting standard care.

Directive for Preventing or Ending the Guilt-Punishment Cycle

Many emergency patients who are suffering from acute pain feel some degree of guilt about the accident that caused the pain. In many instances they know some act of negligence, ignorance, or omission on their part contributed to the accident. When this happens, the pain serves as a just punishment in their mind for this sense of guilt.

If your statements to the patient can bring this idea of guilt to the surface and can then show that enough punishment has already occurred, the resulting relief will diminish the perception of pain.

> *Situation: A twenty-four-year-old woman was involved in a car accident— she has injuries and is crying in pain. The rescuer speaks to her.*

Mary, I may be wrong, but I sense that you are blaming yourself a little for this. Even if there was something you could have done to avoid this, don't you think that what has happened is punishment enough? Good, now let's get on with fixing you up!

Relatable emotions include fear or anger. ("That really scared you, didn't it? You don't think that driver really meant to run you off the road. They probably swerved to miss a deer.") Forgiveness is the treatment of anger.

Directive to Increase the Patient's Sense of Control

The more helpless an emergency patient feels, the more likely they will suffer from pain. The more the rescuer can empower the patient, rather than make them feel the role of victim, the more control they will have of their comfort.[3] The expression of suffering is a way of calling out for help. Whenever you can involve the patient in treating the injury, this sense of helplessness can be reduced. However, when you give a directive that gives the patient some control over the actual pain, a significant improvement can be gained.

An effective directive for giving the patient direct control over the pain can be patterned after the following.

> *Situation: A twenty-eight-year-old female was hiking and has badly twisted her ankle. She is experiencing extreme discomfort.*

Susan, the distress you are experiencing is your body's way of telling you something is wrong. But the signal doesn't have to be as loud as it is for it to reach you. In fact, you can control the volume of the signal while at the same time telling us when we are helping and when we're not. Just imagine that there are colored electrical wires running from your ankle to a light bulb in your brain. Between your ankle and the light in your brain is a dimmer switch that dims or brightens the light. When messages from your ankle head up to the light to indicate your discomfort, you can intervene to control the intensity of the signal. Just to see how easily this works, go ahead and *begin to dim* the light a little now. Good. Now you maintain control with the dimmer to whatever level you need to let us know what is happening.

Direct the Patient to Understand a More Important Priority Than the Injury

In some medical emergencies, there is an urgent need to remove the patient from the scene as quickly as possible. When this occurs, the patient's perception of pain can be changed by getting them to recognize the more significant threat. For example, a fighter will likely ignore most pain that comes with the trauma of the event until the fight is over.

> *Situation: A hiker has broken her leg on a steep, remote mountain trail. Access by helicopter is impossible, and the cold night is approaching. Paramedics have to maneuver the gurney down over rocks and ravines. The task will be almost impossible after dark.*

Joanne, I know how terribly uncomfortable this is for you. However, I want you to help us out as best you can by remaining as still and as quiet as possible. If we don't get you off this mountain before dark, we're all going to be in trouble.

> *You should be cautioned that this type of directive should only be used with a patient in pain whose injury itself is not life-threatening.* Even in such a case, a favorable outcome should be implied, although it is made contingent on their cooperating with the rescuers.

Guide the Patient Toward Healing, Comfortable Images

Directives that help the patient visualize ideas or things that would reduce pain are very effective. What these may be is limited only by your (or the patient's) imagination.

> *Situation: A sixteen-year-old male was riding a horse alongside another horse that kicked him in the shin and fractured his tibia. The boy does not have a good tolerance for pain and continues to complain vehemently. He describes the pain as being sharp and piercing, as though a knife were being jabbed into the bone. Good rapport exists between him and the paramedic, however, and positive expectations have been encouraged.*

Danny, as I wrap this cotton bandage around your leg and the cardboard splint, I want you to close your eyes for a moment and visualize the cotton is so thick and so matted that nothing could pierce through it. When you see that image, next see a sharp knife jabbing at the area, but it can't get through to your leg. You feel the pressure as it jabs into the cotton, but you are much more able to stand this amount of discomfort. Good. When you reach your tolerance level for this dull discomfort, see the knife being withdrawn from the cotton and notice the feeling of relief. Good. Now, Danny, on your way to the hospital you can repeat this process whenever you need to. Just imagine more and more cotton being wrapped around your leg and notice the decrease in discomfort and the increase in comfort. The extra energy you have can now be used to speed up the healing. And remember, don't be mad at that old horse anymore—he wasn't aiming at you.

A second example of the use of guided imagery to reduce the pain experience is seen in the case of an acute abdomen patient. Acute abdomen problems such as appendicitis, peptic ulcer, kidney infection, and so on can cause severe localized pain. Treatment in the field is limited to the anticipation of shock and efforts to transport to the hospital as quickly as possible. Since the patient's knowledge of interior anatomy is usually less than what is known about external anatomy, there is often more confusion and fear about what is going on. Guided imagery can replace fearful, counterproductive images with images that can help the healing process.

> Situation: *A forty-seven-year-old male with a history of peptic ulcers is complaining of extreme pain in the lower right quadrant of the abdomen. During transport, the paramedic utilizes guided imagery with the patient. He speaks matter-of-factly about the use of guided imagery.*

Mr. Vaughn, are you familiar with how the use of mental imagery can redirect certain biochemical processes in the body? Well, it's very effective. We'll be at the hospital in about ten minutes and in that time we can do quite a bit to not only make you more comfortable but also to enhance the healing process and to help your body respond wonderfully to the doctor's treatment later on.

What I'd like you to do is close your eyes, and as you do, notice the immediate increase in comfort. Now, just allow that feeling of increased comfort to increase even more. As it does, notice that you *are beginning* to relax the muscles around your abdomen a little more and that this also increases the sense of comfort. Good. Now I want you to imagine that a crew of special miniature workers that are going down into your stomach to fix the problems that are causing you discomfort. See them going down to fix a sort of protective seal that is in need of repair, and that is allowing stomach acids to get into the stomach lining. *What kind of tools do you think they could use to fix that seal?* [In most instances the patient will offer an idea, such as a special glue, and so on. If not, suggest your own creative imagery.] Good. Now just begin to see this miniature crew working very efficiently as they caulk around the broken seal with the soft, jellylike sealant. And as they do, notice that less stomach acid is allowed to get into the damaged area. OK, it's beginning to work. Just keep on with the work. Soon we'll be at the hospital and whatever treatments you get will serve as a help to the miniature workers!

Give Directives That Shift the Patient's Attention to Another Time and Place

Directives can be used to shift the patient's orientation to a time or place when the pain was not experienced. By drawing attention to a happy memory or thought, the mind cannot pay as close attention to the pain messages.

> *Situation: A thirty-year-old male was using a blowtorch to cut through an empty oil drum to make a barbecue. Fumes remaining in the drum were ignited, and the resultant explosion lacerated and burned the man seriously. During treatment, the first responder attempts to reorient to a different time and place.*

I'll bet you can imagine someplace you'd rather be than here. As a matter of fact, go ahead and do that now while we get you bandaged up. Think of your favorite place. When you are there in your mind's eye, look around and notice all the things there are to notice. Listen to the sounds. Feel the good feelings. There might even be a special aroma you can smell. When you are really experiencing that place, let me know by raising your index finger. Good.

Induce a Relaxation Response

During an emergency, the nervous system accelerates heart rate, respiration, and blood supply to the muscles. Even after the real danger is over, the continuation of these responses tends to keep the patient feeling a sense of danger and pain from the injury. If a relaxation response can be attained, these reactions become reversed. When heart rate, muscle tension, and circulation are relaxed, the patient often feels freedom from pain even in the middle of an emergency.

Since the idea of relaxation during an emergency is likely to be seen as being unrealistic to the patient, the relaxation response is best achieved when it is associated with a specific realistic reason—for example, having the patient relax so that an accurate reading can be taken with the blood pressure cuff; or a patient with angina pain is likely to understand that by slowing their heart rate they can better fill their coronary arteries. Once a realistic association is made, directives for relaxation are likely to be accepted. Note that direct suggestions for relaxation can be tied in with directives described in the preceding section.

> *Situation: A twenty-two-year-old male hiker dislocated his left shoulder during a slip and fall on the trail. He is ten miles from the nearest access point to emergency help. One of his companions runs for help. The second stays*

with him. Trained in these procedures of communication, he proceeds to help his friend:

Pete, while we are waiting for John to get help, I want to tell you what I know that can make you more comfortable. The terrible discomfort you are feeling is happening because your arm and shoulder muscles are tight and are straining the tendons and ligaments that have been stretched. If you relax the entire arm and shoulder, those relaxed muscles would ease the strain. [In some cases the muscles will relax so much the shoulder can easily be relocated, even though this is not recommended for paramedics to attempt.]

Now, when I count to three, I want you to take a deep breath and then let it all the way out. As you exhale, notice the muscles in your arm and shoulder relaxing. Then, they will continue to relax more with each exhalation.

Give the Patient a Way to Change the Intensity of Pain

When the pain experience cannot be removed, it is relatively easy to help the patient modify it. An easy way to do this is by using a pain scale, having the patient locate where on the scale the pain is, then encouraging them to go lower on the scale.

> *Situation: A twenty-eight-year-old female injured her knee during a marathon run. Swelling and pain are severe.*

Susan, in a moment I want you to describe the level of *discomfort* in your knee on a scale of 1 to 10. Let the number 10 be the most discomfort you can imagine, like a knife jabbing in your knee or a red hot iron, and let the number 1 be a mild pressure like someone just touching you with their finger. *You may be surprised* to see how easily you can change the level, upwards or downwards, from where you are now. I'll show you. Please tell me where you are now with your knee on that scale. [The patient says 8 or 9.] OK, now, just for a moment, move it down and tell me where you moved it to. [The patient says 6 or 7.] Good. Would you be willing to move it back to 8 or 9 for just a moment? (Patient either agrees or prefers not to. If he does not want to, that is fine. If she does, it increases her sense of control, and she may next move it all the way down to 3 or 4.)

In the case of a child, this same technique may be used with the assistance of the Wong-Baker FACES pain chart. A child can point to the color or facial expression that helps them control the pain. This visual chart may also be helpful when treating adults because adults who exaggerate their pain level with the number system may be expressing fear. Looking at a chart gives your patient an opportunity to re-focus on a tangible representation of their pain. According to a pediatric study on this scale, the Wong–Baker FACES pain chart was found to be reliable in measuring pain as an element separate from fear.[4]

Give a Direct Suggestion for Comfort and Pain Relief

For extremely frightened emergency patients, direct suggestions can be quick and effective—for example, "The discomfort in your head is gone," or "When I count to three, your head will feel clear and comfortable." The risk with such directives, however, is that they may not work. You are not a wizard who can speak things into being. It is only your prompting that works to guide the patient into a healing disposition. But, the patient may not be ready for your directives. When this happens, you lose a little rapport, and you might even lose some self-confidence. Nonetheless, there will be times when such directives are appropriate.

> *Situation: A forty-two year old female was pinned behind the wheel of her car with multiple injuries. Two other cars were involved in the accident and there are three injured people in each car. The female driver's chest is pushed hard against the steering wheel, and she is hysterically screaming about her pain. The rescuer and her partner are involved in assigning triage priorities while waiting for more help. The woman's screaming is frightening other patients on the scene and is preventing the rescuer from examining her condition effectively. When speaking to hysterical patients, it is often helpful to place a confident, firm, but gentle hand on a shoulder and speak softly into their ear. Patients tend to concentrate better on words that are whispered in their ears when in this condition. The rescuer speaks to the woman.*

I know how much you are hurting and how scared and maybe even angry you are, but the *worst is over now.* Soon we'll have you and your friends out of here, but we need your help. Will you help us? Good [whether or not the patient actually agrees]. Now, first, you need to breathe easier. When I count to three, you'll notice how much easier and more relaxed it will be for you to breathe. One, two, three. Good.

Give a Directive for Glove Anesthesia

Another kind of directive that can be given to alleviate pain is called *glove anesthesia.* This refers to a technique used in medical hypnosis to prepare patients for surgery when chemical anesthesia is not desired.[5] Although it is a direct type of suggestion, it gives the patient a feeling of control over their pain. When time permits, an emergency patient can be taught how to use glove anesthesia to control their discomfort at will.

> *Situation: A twenty-four-year-old male is a patient after being assaulted. He has multiple contusions (bruises). He is conscious. Whenever paramedics try to move him, he resists and complains of pain. None of the injuries appear to be life-threatening, and the rescuer has managed to establish a positive*

rapport with him. The rescuer decides to utilize glove anesthesia because it will give control back to this patient.

Arnold, I'm going to give you a powerful tool that you can use *any way you choose to help yourself feel better.* In fact, you can reduce the discomfort and increase the healing at any particular place on your body where you need to. OK, look at your fingertips for a moment and notice how you can make the tips of them numb as though they were all sprayed with Novocain. Touch each fingertip with your thumb and notice how the feeling is going away, as though you were touching the rubber fingers of a mannequin or a doll. Good. You can allow that *feeling of numbness* to spread up your fingers and into your hand until your entire hand begins to feel numb, or it may feel cold as though it were being dipped into ice water.

Now, whenever you are ready, you can use this hand to transfer this cool or numb feeling to any part of your body that would benefit you. For example, go ahead and touch the bump on your forehead and notice how it also becomes cool or numb. Notice, too, how much more comfortable that feels. Arnold, we are going to put you on the gurney now. Whenever you feel discomfort, just touch that part of your body where you need it the most.

Masking the Pain

Pain serves a purpose. It is a warning that something is wrong. Once the warning is heeded, however, the pain becomes unnecessary. Emotional factors such as fear and other learned perceptions usually maintain pain and suffering until these things no longer serve a constructive purpose. However, to the degree that first responders and emergency physicians need to know what is wrong with the patient, it is not desirable for *all* of the patient's pain to go away.

The above directives will not usually cause all the pain to disappear. The patient will be more comfortable and may stop suffering, but they will still be able to communicate about the source of the pain. However, particularly responsive patients may mask over the pain completely. For this reason, each directive you give should include a suggestion for the patient to keep just enough discomfort at the injury site so that they can continue to tell you the effect of the treatment and so that they can tell the same to the doctor. This suggestion has the added benefit of giving control over the pain back to the patient.

Exercise

You have a patient complaining of severe pain in their fractured elbow. Describe exactly what you would say (and how you would say it) to help relieve the pain. Remember, to use the word "discomfort" instead of "pain."

Notes

1 Jensen, M. (October, 2008). The neurophysiology of pain perception and hypnotic analgesia: Implications for clinical practice. *American Journal of Clinical Hypnosis*, 51(2), 123–148.

2 Keller, D.M. (July, 2020). Hypnosis may relieve pain, cut reliance on morphine at atrial flutter ablation. *Medscape*. https://www.medscape.com/viewarticle/933577

3 Elmqvist, C., Fridlund, B., & Ekebergh, M. (2008). More than medical treatment: The patient's first encounter with prehospital emergency care. *International Emergency Nursing*, 16(3), 185–192.

4 Garra, G., Singer, A.J., Domingo, A., & Thode Jr, H.C. (2013). The Wong-Baker pain FACES scale measures pain, not fear. *Pediatric Emergency Care*, 29(1), 17–20.

5 Cozzolino, M., Celia, G., Rossi, K.L., & Rossi, E.L. (2020). Hypnosis as sole anesthesia for dental removal in a patient with multiple chemical sensitivity. *International Journal of Clinical and Experimental Hypnosis*, 68(3), 371–383.

11 Stopping Bleeding

This chapter deals with the patient's ability to follow directives to stop their own bleeding, as an adjunct to standard medical procedures, such as direct pressure and bandaging.

As far back as 1975, physicians referred to case histories that show hypnosis can control massive bleeding.[1,2,3] Dentists and physicians have been using or teaching hypnosis to hemophiliacs since the 1960s according to the Journal of the American Medical Association.[4]

Beyond specific evidence about the control of bleeding in peer-reviewed journals, we can infer from studies that show hypnosis can reduce anxiety and blood pressure, that its effect on bleeding would be significant. The variable amount of bleeding from similar wounds in different emergency patients may be another indication of psychological control. One person's laceration may bleed intensely. Another's may not bleed at all. Often, a patient does not start bleeding from an injury until after the paramedics arrive and start talking about blood.

The ability of some individuals to voluntarily control bleeding is well documented. Numerous surgical procedures involving hypnotic suggestion or acupuncture have been accomplished with unusually small amounts of bleeding. One study, described in the BBC film, *Can Your Mind Control Your Body?* showed a major reduction in bleeding during dental surgery with 200 hemophiliacs. Without hypnotic suggestion, the hemophiliacs required from five to thirty-five transfusions of blood. With hypnotic suggestion they required from two to three.

It is not known precisely how thoughts or directives physiologically decrease hemorrhage. It seems to relate to constriction of blood vessels and coagulation of blood as well as to some other basic biochemical changes.

David Cheek, M.D., an obstetrician and a pioneer in the use of medical hypnosis, has speculated that the sudden cessation of arteriolar and venous bleeding is due to a high outpouring of epinephrine followed by the relaxation of muscles surrounding the injury. Epinephrine does increase the coagulation speed of blood. But, typically rebound fibrinolytic activity causes secondary bleeding.

DOI: 10.4324/9781003430261-14

Perhaps confident directives to relax and stop bleeding inhibit internal messages to send fibrinolysins to the injured area so that the initial response to the epinephrine is maintained. Since standard field treatments are minimal for internal bleeding, whether, from a bleeding ulcer, a broken rib, a closed fracture, or a bad bruise, these emergency hypnosis directives for such injuries might also result in saving lives.

Whatever the processes involved, directives to stop bleeding can be very effective at the emergency scene. The following case studies illustrate the phrasing you may want to use.

Situation: A thirty-four-year-old woman was thrown from a vehicle in a multiple-car accident and is bleeding from a small artery in the lip and from a deep laceration in the scalp by the time help arrives. After taking a moment to appraise the situation and gain self confidence, the paramedic puts his thumb on the woman's forehead to get her attention and says, "Listen to me. You are OK. Stop that bleeding now." The woman stops her bleeding, and the paramedic goes to look at another patient. A bystander yells out, "You'd better get those people away from the car before it blows up—there's gasoline leaking!" At that point, the first patient starts crying and her bleeding begins again. The paramedic quiets the bystanders, assures everyone that there is going to be no explosion and returns to the patient, again placing his thumb on her forehead. "Listen to me. The worst is over. Now stop that bleeding. You did it before and you can do it again." Again, the woman's bleeding stops and arriving paramedics begin direct pressure bandaging and stabilization procedures.

Situation: A twenty-two-year-old male bicyclist not wearing a helmet suffered a scalp laceration when his bicycle spun out coming down a steep hill. Upon arrival, the fire fighters find the patient alert and completely oriented. He is badly shaken, however, and frightened enough to be in an alternative state of consciousness as evidenced by his hyper-suggestible, smooth facial expression and fixed eye staring. Bleeding has stopped, but the hair is matted with blood and the wound is filled with road dirt and debris.

Bill, you can start and stop your own bleeding by simply concentrating on turning it on or off. We need to clean some of the debris out of your wound, and it would help us if you would go ahead and allow it to bleed again just for a moment. Go ahead and do that now. Good, that helps.

While the paramedic cleans out the debris with a sterilized 4-by-4inch pad, the patient begins oozing blood that helps with the process. After about ten seconds the wound is prepared for bandaging. Direct pressure bandaging is applied, and Bill is asked to stop the bleeding again:

OK, Bill, we've got the wound clean and we can bandage it now. When I count to three, I want you to stop the bleeding again.

Situation: A fifty-four-year-old male with a history of stomach ulcers has vomited blood while at the beach. His pulse is thready, his skin is clammy, and his eyes are dull. The patient states that he is thirsty and that he is afraid he is going to die. While the two arriving lifeguards administer oxygen, place the patient in the shock position, and wait for the ambulance, one of them has managed to gain rapport and build expectations for a positive future using several strategies outlined in the previous chapters. The lifeguard is now ready to give a directive to get the patient to stop the internal bleeding.

Mr. Edwards, as you know, your stomach is probably bleeding again. You can stop that bleeding yourself, and I'm going to tell you how. I want you to imagine, just imagine, that you have sent a crew of workers down into your stomach to patch up the places where it is bleeding. Will you do that? Just imagine them *any way you choose*, but see how quickly and efficiently they are able to patch up your stomach and stop the bleeding. Good. That image is already working. Your blood pressure is beginning to stabilize. Now, I want you to continue with those images all the way to the hospital.

Situation: A six-year old child crawls into a kennel with five sled dogs. Playing with her they cause cuts on several parts of her body, sufficient to cause blood flow. Seeing her blood she begins to scream. Her parents, who had been talking to the mailman with their backs to the child, turned and quickly removed the child while the mailman called the fire department. When the EMT/firefighter team arrived, the parents were telling the child she would be OK and that the cuts were not that bad and that the dogs did not want to hurt her. However, the child continued screaming and was having difficulty breathing. As one of the EMTs ran back to the truck to get the oxygen bottle, the other kneeled down in front of the child and spoke:

Oh my gosh, look at all the blood! That must be scary to see your bright red blood all over your arms and legs. But you are really doing a good job of using that beautiful red blood to clean out all the dirt so you can go ahead and stop it now and help me finish cleaning you up with these clean white gauze pads.

The bleeding and the screaming stopped before the oxygen bottle arrived and was not needed.

Note that research studies on hypnosis relating to autonomic nervous system control of such functions as bleeding are often controversial because findings are not consistent. This is the case for blood flow control. For example, one study[5] wanted to see if a subject in a laboratory setting instructed to reduce bleeding time in one arm and to let the other arm bleed, could not control bleeding time. The researchers found they were not able to slow bleeding time. A variety of reasons may be considered. For examples, it could have been the rapport between the hypnotizer and the hypnotized. It could be the psychological conflict about letting one arm bleed, while stopping the other. It could be the individual simply did not go into sufficient hypnosis in the lab setting, etc. It could even relate to pre-study disbelief that the subject could do it. In any case, the evidence is strong scientifically and anecdotally for the potential of blood control in the medical emergency patient.

Exercises

1   What strategy did the EMT employ in the last situation?
2   Using the case of the 54-year-old male with a bleeding ulcer from this chapter, create your own directive using descriptive metaphors to create images that could help stop the bleeding.
3   Imagine and practice how you would craft your communication when interacting with a patient with an arterial bleed versus a superficial bleed.
4   What types of imagery might be helpful when directing a patient to stop bleeding?

Notes

1   Clawson, T.A. Jr., & Swade, R.H. (1975). The hypnotic control of blood flow and pain: The cure of warts and the potential for the use of hypnosis in the treatment of cancer. *American Journal of Clinical Hypnosis,* 17(3), 160–169. https://doi.org/10. 1080/00029157.1975.10403735
2   Kihlstrom, J.F. (2004). *Encyclopedia of Applied Psychology.* https://www.sciencedirect. com/topics/medicine-and-dentistry/hypnosis
3   Owen, S., Surman, M.D., & Lee Baer, Ph.D. (2008) *Massachusetts General Hospital Comprehensive Clinical Psychiatry.* https://www.sciencedirect.com/topics/ medicine-and-dentistry/hypnosis
4   Martin, J. (1983). Hypnosis may reduce hemophiliac's blood needs. *JAMA.* https:// jamanetwork.com/journals/jama/article-abstract/388200
5   Hopkins, M.B., Jordan, J.M., & Lunday, R.M. (Originally published 1989). The effects of hypnosis and of imagery on bleeding time. *International Journal of Clinical and Experimental Hypnosis,* 39(3), 134–139.

12 Cardiovascular Emergencies

The rescuer's ability to calm and reassure the cardiac or stroke patient can prevent secondary attacks and stabilize vital signs. This chapter describes how to use hypnotic communication with a cardiac patient at various levels of severity. This is followed by a discussion and sample approach on how one might communicate with a stroke patient.

Thoughts and emotions have a significant influence on our hearts. States of anxiety can raise blood pressure and heart rate. Relaxation can lower them. People can learn to control these functions voluntarily to a significant degree, though they are usually considered to be involuntary nervous system responses. For example, yoga masters have demonstrated the ability to drastically raise or lower their pulse and blood pressure, as have students training with biofeedback equipment. Similarly, meditation classes have been extremely effective in helping hypertensive patients manage their blood pressure without drugs.[1]

Treating or Preventing Shock

During medical emergencies, the action of the heart and blood vessels is affected by a variety of conditions. Such conditions can cause the patient's nervous system to dilate or contract the size of the arteries and veins, thus raising or lowering blood pressure. If the blood pressure is too high, vessels can rupture. If too low, vital organs may be seriously damaged and life-threatening shock may occur. Since so many conditions, from anxiety and blood loss to infection and bee stings, can lead to shock, treating for shock is always a first aid consideration for most medical emergencies.

Preventing or treating shock has generally meant repositioning the patient so blood can return to the heart more easily (preventing, further loss of blood and body heat). Administering oxygen or providing airway management is another obvious priority. However, none of these procedures take full advantage of the tremendous capability of the patient's own autonomic nervous system. Since the adaptive ability of the nervous system is often compromised by misdirected or overactive thoughts, new directives can help restore equilibrium in the same

DOI: 10.4324/9781003430261-15

way that falling down can restore normal perfusion in the person who has fainted (psychogenic shock).

It is relatively easy to give patients directives for raising or lowering heart rate and blood pressure, once confidence, rapport, and expectations have been gained. It should be noted that individuals can control either function independently of the other. In other words, a patient may lower their heart rate without changing blood pressure or vice versa. The medic will want to monitor both.

> *Situation: A fifty-three-year-old female is showing signs and symptoms of shock, including a weak and rapid pulse rate of 120 and a low blood pressure of 100/60. Her skin is clammy and pale. She is conscious, and she tells the rescuer she has had severe nausea and diarrhea for several days. The rescuer talks to the patient on the way to the hospital.*

Martha, you've lost lots of fluid, and it has been difficult for your heart to pump oxygenated blood to all the parts of your body. Just imagine a garden hose with a small volume of water running through it. Notice how slowly the water drips out of the end. But if you narrow the size of the opening, the water comes out faster. Your body can adjust the size of your blood vessels to compensate for the loss of water. Go ahead now and allow your body to make those adjustments so that oxygenated blood can be carried to all the parts of your body that need it, especially your brain, your heart, your lungs, and your kidneys. Just begin to feel how these organs are right now being given adequate amounts of oxygen-rich blood.

Research has shown that individuals can learn to direct increases in blood flow to specific locations in the body. For example, one study proved that a "single 30-minute hypnosis session decreased pain intensity" because the hypnosis "increased peripheral vasodilation during both the anticipation and experience of pain in patients with sickle-cell disease that leads to sympathetic nervous system dysfunction."[2]

Elmer and Alice Green of the Menninger Foundation also taught patients to vasodilate vessels in their autogenic feedback training, a form of hypnosis, so the hand where patients increased hand temperatures have increased by as much as 25 degrees Fahrenheit.[3] By asking emergency patients who may be going into shock to concentrate on blood flowing to those vital organs that cannot lack perfusion for very long, cardiovascular responses may enhance survivability until more technical, medical procedures can be applied at the hospital.

Acute Myocardial Infarction (Heart Attack)

The mind-body connection seems particularly obvious when referring to injury to the heart muscle. Even the traditional poetic metaphor, as in "You have broken my heart," points to this connection. Theories that suggest that some personality types are more susceptible to acute myocardial infarction (AMI), or heart attacks, also infer that the health of the heart is linked to mental processes. And, there is little doubt that emotional stress and anxiety can significantly influence heart function and blood pressure.

Once a heart attack has occurred, it is likely that mental considerations influence physiological responses. Some studies show that deaths can result, not from the initial heart attack, but from secondary attacks that relate to anxiety about the first one. The extremely frightening nature of having a heart attack makes the patient extremely responsive to proper communication from attending rescuers. The nervous system remains capable of coordinating heart fibers, increasing or decreasing heart rate, and reducing inflammation in heart tissue. Directives that create appropriate nervous system image-responses like these can be lifesaving.

When a patient presents a cardiac emergency with symptoms such as chest pain that may radiate to the jaw arm or back, difficulty breathing, diaphoresis, or vertigo. The standard care usually is administering aspirin, nitroglycerine and/or other pain medication, along with nonemergency transportation to the hospital. However, hypnotic communication can be very useful. To cite an *International Journal of Cardiology and Heart Vasculature* article published in 2020:

> From a pathophysiological point of view, the effect of hypnosis on cardiac arrhythmias is still little understood, although the modulation of the autonomic nervous system (ANS) seems to play a key role…Hypnosis is effective in the reduction of anxiety and psychological stress, and is capable of influencing both the hypothalamic–pituitaryadrenal axis, and modulating the ANS by increasing the parasympathetic tone and decreasing the sympathetic tone…
>
> hypnosis is still underused in clinical practice with misconceptions and misunderstandings still standing in the way.[4]

Situation: A forty-six-year-old male with a history of mild hypertension has suffered a heart attack. When the responder arrives on the scene, the patient is conscious and describes a substernal pain characterized as "squeezing" and radiating to his jaw and left arm. The pain has lasted for over an hour. Heart rate is 140. The 12-Lead EKG shows ST elevation in V3 and V4.

Mr. Davis, it appears that you have had a minor heart attack affecting the anterior part of your heart. This is the front part of your heart *(touching patient)* I know how frightening the feeling you have now seems, but the worst is over. Your body is now trying to regain a homeostasis or balance, and if you do what I say, I can help you regain that status more quickly. Will you do as I say? (The patient acknowledges in the affirmative.) Good.

Up to this point the rescuer has projected confidence, given the patient positive expectations for the immediate future, and, through the direct contract strategy, gained positive rapport. Remember to speak calmly and professionally.

One of the common aspects of acute myocardial infarction is a feeling of impending doom. If this is allowed to continue, the arrhythmia may produce disorganized ventricular activity followed by fibrillation and death.

Although telling the patient that his body is now trying to regain homeostasis or balance may in itself be a sufficient indirect suggestion to regain a normal heart rhythm, at this point a more specific directive can be helpful.

OK, Mr. Davis, I want you to concentrate on breathing in this fresh, pure oxygen from the mask and send it to your heart to help the uninjured muscle fibers carry on the efficient, organized work of pumping that oxygenated blood through your body. Now I really want you to imagine, in whatever way you choose, that those heart muscle fibers are regaining their composure and are beginning to work smoothly again. You might imagine a team leader down there directing the group of muscle fibers to work in an efficient, coordinated way, easily compensating the tissues that were injured. As you do this, notice that you are beginning to slow your heart rate down. Since the team is working so efficiently now, fewer beats are required to get the work done. Good. You're doing well. I have spoken with the doctor, and they are expecting you.

Cardiac Arrest

A percentage of cardiac emergencies will be patients who are going into or already in cardiac arrest. This means the heart has stopped beating altogether or is in a state of completely disorganized quivering, called fibrillation. Other situations might involve a patient with extremely low blood pressure or pulseless electrical activity (PEA). The chance to save such a patient exists only if treatments can be administered within a short time, usually about three to four minutes. In many cases, immediate initiation of cardiopulmonary resuscitation (CPR) has been responsible for patient survival of cardiac arrest. CPR in itself, however, is comparatively inefficient, and success rates for reviving patients of cardiac arrest are not high. Perhaps if internal mental forces could be tapped during CPR, more effective results could be achieved.

The aforementioned article has many citations supporting hypnotic interventions for cardiac problems, but we only have anecdotal evidence for severe witnessed heart attacks that require CPR or electric shock. This comes from patients who survived and looked up the contact information for rescuers, thanking them for the words they heard during the event despite being apparently unconscious. Unconscious individuals continue to be aware of what they construe to be meaningful sounds. Dr. Dabney Ewin has reported responses in heart rate and blood pressure to verbal commands in surgical patients under general anesthesia. If the nervous system can be directed to regain normal heart rhythm in a conscious patient, it may be able to stop fibrillation or even restart heartbeat during asystole.[5]

Stroke

Stroke patients may not be able to speak to you at the emergency scene. Or, some may experience expressive aphasia that prevents them from getting the words out as intended. You must look for signs that indicate that the patient is responding to your communication. Such signs could be as subtle as the blink of an eye. One way to set up a communicative structure is to ask the patient to answer yes or no questions by raising the second and third fingers of one hand to indicate one finger for yes and the other finger for no. The ideomotor reflex (described earlier in the text) will thus be activated and serve three functions. First, it provides an immediate opportunity for two-way communication; second, it gives the stroke patient a sense of control in spite of the debilitating nature of the injury; and third, it helps create a special rapport between you and the victim.

When an ischemic stroke occurs, an interruption of cerebral blood flow damages a portion of the brain. This impairs some biochemical or physiological function that was initiated at the site of injury. Many times we can notice symptoms of a stroke but not know the part of the brain affected or how it is being affected without getting a brain scan. For example, some strokes are caused by a bleed in the brain while others are caused by a clot that prevents blood flow to part of the brain. We have already seen how hypnosis can influence blood flow.

Although we know very little about the brain, we do know that the majority of brain cells are not activated regularly. We also know that certain portions of the brain can learn to take over functions usually controlled by other areas.[6] These patients developed new internal sensory circuits from the brain to the affected motor neurons.[7] As a result, normal functioning returned. Whether this can happen spontaneously in a stroke patient during the first hour of trauma is unknown, however, using hypnotic language to influence blood flow to the brain may help.

> *Situation: A sixty-eight-year-old female has difficulty with speech and partial paralysis on the left side of the body. While standard first aid procedures are being initiated, the rescuer is speaking calmly and confidently to the patient.*

Mrs. Bradley, I know that you can hear me, and I know that you are very frightened about what has happened to you. You may have had a blood vessel injury in your head that has temporarily immobilized some of your muscles. While your brain figures out how to compensate, we are going to help you by ... [Describe interventions being used such as IV, O2, and EKG as well as preparations with the hospital to get to a CT scanner and Neurologist] In a few minutes I'm going to show you how you can begin using the uninjured portions of your brain to assist your breathing and your swallow reflex. Right now I want you to just close your eyes and imagine being in some favorite resting place of yours. The ambulance is on its way, and things are being made ready for you at the hospital. Now, if you can understand what I am saying, I want you to indicate that by raising the index finger on your left hand. You don't have to raise it very much, just a little will do. Go ahead and do that now. [Patient responds.] Good.

Now, go ahead to that special restful place while we put you on the ambulance bed and get you ready for our drive to the hospital. Let me know by moving that finger when you are at that place in your mind's eye. [Again, the patient responds.] Good.

> *At this point the rescuer can attempt to give a more profound directive that might allow the patient to regain control of some vital function, such as breathing regularly, that might be at risk for further complications or failure. The rescuer has built up expectations for it with the phrase, "while your brain figures out how to compensate."*

OK, Mrs. Bradley, your body is already beginning to heal from your stroke in its own way. The doctors are waiting for you at the hospital. Until we get there, however, there is much you can do to get other portions of your brain to help you control your breathing. It won't be easy because you have been doing it one way for a long time, but if you are willing, try, and I'm sure it will help. Are you willing to try? [Patient responds positively.] Good. Now, all I want you to do is to notice that you have different ways to signal your chest muscles to move and to signal your diaphragm to move. Experiment until you are able to take a little breath on your own.

If vital functions are not in jeopardy, the rescuer will probably not choose to direct the patient to learn how to activate a paralyzed muscle group at the emergency scene. This is best reserved for the physical therapist. However, if directives can help save the patient's life, this approach is certainly worth trying during the extra time that is available while waiting for the ambulance or during transport to the hospital.

Note that, for both heart attacks and strokes, it is often just as important to use effective communication with the patient's family as it is with the patient. For guidelines relating to this, see Chapter 17, "Psychological Crisis."

True or False?

1 It is possible that the inability to calm and reassure victims of heart attacks may be responsible for secondary heart attacks.
2 It is possible that an unconscious patient on whom you are doing CPR might hear your words and respond to them.
3 Patients can be directed to control such autonomic nervous system functions as pulse rate and blood pressure.
4 Patients who have expressive aphasia are not able to benefit from hypnotic communication.

Notes

1 Heart Health. (June, 2020). Meditation and a relaxation technique to lower blood pressure. *Harvard Medical School Education Online*. https://www.health.harvard.edu/heart-health/meditation-and-a-relaxation-technique-to-lower-blood-pressure

2 Bhatt, R.R., Martin, S.R., Evans, S., Lung, K., Coates, T.D., Zeitzer, L.K. and Tsa, J.C. (July, 2017). The effect of hypnosis on pain and peripherifal blood flow in sickle-cell disease. *Journal of Pain Research*, 10, 1635–1644. Republished by pubmed at https://www.ncbi.nlm.nih.gov/pmc/articles/PMC5529094/

3 Green, E., & Green, A. (1977). *Beyond Biofeedback*. Knoll Publishing, 35–36.

4 Berner, A. (February, 2022). Arrhythmia conversion to sinus rhythm during hypnosis. https://www.ncbi.nlm.nih.gov/pmc/articles/PMC8724937/

5 Kotsovolis, G. (2009). Awareness during anesthesia: Hos sure can we be that the patient is sleeping indeed? *Hippoktratia*, 13(2), 83–89.

6 Li, R., Mukadam, N., & Kiran, S. (2022). Functional MRI evidence for reorganization of language networks after stroke. *Handbook of Clinical Neurology*, 185, 131–150.

7 Siegel, J.S., Shulman, G.L., & Corbetta, M. (2022). Mapping correlated neurological deficits after stroke to distributed brain networks. *Brain Structure and Function*, 227(9), 3173–3187.

13　Hypnotic Treatment for Burns

This chapter discusses how proper directives for burn victims has the potential to influence the nervous system so as to reduce inflammatory processes. It refers to thermal, chemical, and sunburn injuries.

Despite most studies relating to the effectiveness of hypnotic communication on burn injuries being largely anecdotal, significant studies are proving it can lead to healing and prevent deeper levels of burn damage. "The acute, identifiable nature of burn care procedures and the emotional state of patients in trauma care both provide an often receptive setting for the use of this intervention."[1]

A rationale for why hypnosis can work follows this logic:

1　Hypnosis can reduce burn pain[2]
2　Pain is caused by inflammation.[3]
3　Hypnosis can reduce inflammation.[4]

Burn injuries are common medical emergencies. Using our mnemonic, CREDIBLE, with burn victims can result in dramatic effects. With proper communication at the emergency scene the inflammatory response of a burn injury, along with fever, pain, and blistering, can be drastically reduced. In one case Four Arrows attended, a patient suffering a deep second-degree burn recovered 12 days without surgery, significant pain, or disfiguration. Such burns usually require 6 to 8 weeks of painful recovery before healing. The patient was a 32-year-old male who was burned by an acetylene torch when the hose broke. (Acetylene burns at three thousand degrees Celsius.) The patient was asked to imagine clean snow falling on the wound, allowing the coolness to heal it while cool towels were placed over the wound. Although the heat from the torch was sufficient to vaporize the patient's shirt and charcoal his skin, no pain medication was necessary. The patient returned to work the next day. In just eight days, the charcoaled skin began peeling off and healthy skin was showing beneath it. In twelve days, the wound was healed with no scar tissue or permanent burn scar.

Such benefits of hypnosis have long been known and proven by medical doctors. For example, an old issue of Time Magazine describes a five-person team

DOI: 10.4324/9781003430261-16

from the University of Texas Southwestern Medical School using hypnosis on extremely burned patients. Here are some quotes from the article:[5]

B.W., 24, with second-degree burns covering 45 percent of his body surface, had undergone several unsuccessful skin grafts in 18 months, went from 130 to 90 Ibs because of refusal to eat properly. Skin infections and contractures (contracted-burn scar tissue) made it difficult for him to move his limbs and neck. Within a few days after hypnosis began, he was taking 4,200 calories per day, became cheerful and cooperative. Thanks to improved diet, skin grafts began to "take." Twelve weeks later, B. W., healed, walked out of the hospital.

J.C., 33, suffered 45 percent body-surface burns in a boiler explosion. His dressings could only be changed under anesthesia; he feared moving his painfully burned hands and fingers. The Southwestern team started daily hypnosis; shunning narcotics, the patient obediently began to exercise his hands as instructed every 30 minutes, even in his sleep, until the doctors stopped him with a posthypnotic order.

C.J., 32, suffered from 35 percent burns, started hypnotic treatment only four hours after the injury. As a result, no anesthesia was required to dull pain, even during skin grafts. With a good appetite and exercise, C. J. spent only 18 days in hospital.

The phenomenon of fire walking also illustrates the ability of the body to react to heat in such a way as to diminish pain and inflammation. Studies of fire walkers in Fiji and India indicate that a strong belief system is responsible. In India, fire walking is preceded by a three-week meditation ritual. In Fiji, fire walkers are told from birth that they have been given this special ability. In the United States, the first author and others have successfully walked across 1,500-degree coals, barefoot, using hypnosis. In all cases, some image formed in the mind stopped that part of the burning that triggers the pain and inflammation response. Co-author of this text, Four Arrows, did the fire walk when he was a firefighter/ EMT for Marine County Fire Department. It was aired on ABC news. He walked across the coals twice while in uniform with his pant legs rolled up. Several hours later, while he and his fellow firefighters were watching it on the television, he suddenly popped a blister, presumably from intensely watching his feet on the glowing embers while no longer in a hypnotic state!

Directives for burns that are given within one or two hours after the initial injury call for vasoconstriction to the burn site, *not* vasodilation, so cooling as with the snow image above is recommended. For many burn patients, this kind of modification in the usual physiological and psychological burn response can not only speed recovery and decrease suffering, it can save lives. When burns affect vital tissues or initiate shock, the relatively simple communication strategies that have been presented, combined with directives that produce images of being cool and comfortable can make a significant difference in survivability. This knowledge would be especially useful for fire fighters, for obvious reasons. And, since the effect requires the communication immediately after the injury, first responders have the greatest opportunity for making a difference in treatment outcome.

Situation: A forty-eight-year-old male was driving a tractor when it broke an underground gas pipe, and a spark ignited a jet of gas. The driver sustained 24 percent total body surface second-degree burns. Rescuers are on the scene within fifteen minutes of receiving the call from the man's wife. After initial assessment, sterile dressings are applied to the surface burns; oxygen is administered; sufficient confidence, rapport, and expectations are developed within several minutes of arrival, using several strategies. The rescuer gives the following directive while applying the sterile dressing:

OK Mr. Brown. Do you know how to take care of this burn? (The patient admits that he does not.) Well, I do. But you can help me by thinking some happy thoughts, because, believe it or not, I can treat you better when you do. Now you seem angry about the fact that you didn't know about the gas pipe location before you started work. It seems like an honest mistake to me. Besides, I think you've already been hurt enough with this accident, don't you?

Note that directives to eliminate guilt are especially useful for burn patients since very often the burn is a result of some negligent act. The rescuer continues.

Now, while we are preparing you for transport to the hospital, I want you to close your eyes for |just a moment and imagine that, as I place the sterile gauze on your injuries, I am really packing the entire area in soft, clean snow. Remember what it was like to put your arm into a wall of very soft, very fresh, fallen snow? Notice how cool and comfortable each area is becoming as you see the snow being applied. Good.

The rescuer repeats this kind of image-producing dialogue several times. Remember that repetition helps the subconscious learn, but only up to a point. Generally, repeating the directive three to four times is sufficient. After that, there can be a tendency for the repetitive statement to cause a sense of urgency that activates analytic thinking at the expense of imagery thinking. Thus, after repeating the cool and comfortable imagery several times, the rescuer changes the focus as follows:

Good. Just allow that cool, comfortable feeling to continue on its own while we put you in the ambulance. Just concentrate on your right calf muscle, and see how relaxed it can become if you first tighten the muscle and then relax it. Go ahead and try that now. Good. Now just move that feeling of relaxation up through the rest of your body for the remainder of the ride to the hospital.

Note that the calf muscle is an uninjured part of the body. By focusing the patient's attention on relaxing an uninjured portion of the body, two things are accomplished. First, the directive for keeping the burn injury cool and comfortable until it heals is sealed in the subconscious as the rescuer matter-of-factly goes on to another subject. Second, the relaxation response that comes from tightening, then relaxing, an uninvolved muscle will in itself augment the psychological relaxation that will help calm and reassure the patient during transport.

Besides images of the snow, the rescuer can use images of a cool mist of water, a cool, clean brook, a shady breeze, and so on can be used. Remember to add to your cool-and-comfortable-directives words that imply cleanliness, freshness, and so on. Whenever possible, use the images that the patient tells you best bring about cool and comfortable feelings. This may augment the mind body's natural tendency to heal wounds treated in this manner without risk of infection.

Besides thermal burns, chemical burns and sunburns can also be treated with the cool-and-In the video, "Emergency Hypnosis VOB" that can be viewed on YouTube,[6] Dr. Gerald Kaplan describes the use of this procedure with his son who suffered bad sun exposure after falling asleep at the beach. He directed him to imagine his face remaining cool and comfortable. The next day his face was not burned; however, his ears were. After considering what happened, Dr. Kaplan speculated that his son had not construed his ears to be a part of his face.

Other environmental emergencies due to heat exposure include heat cramps, heat exhaustion, and heat stroke. In each case, the heat regulatory mechanisms are overwhelmed enough to cause a breakdown. While administering standard field treatment for each of these problems, simple directives can slow down or temporarily reverse the breakdown process.

The skin is especially influenced by psychological determinants. Hives, blushing, goose pimpling, and so on are all common emotional reactions. The skin, the largest single organ of the body, also serves to regulate the temperature of the body and to transmit information from the environment to the brain. Nerve endings that lie in the skin perceive and transmit information about heat, cold, pain, pleasure, and so on. As with any illness or injury, an overreactive vicious circle can begin when negative images from past experiences are triggered. Although physical cooling or hydration is extremely important, the capability of psychological cooling should not be neglected.

Situation: A twenty-five-year-old female was hiking on a hot day in a large park. Park personnel were informed that she had fallen down on the trail and was complaining of dizziness and nausea. The rescuer responds and establishes a positive rapport. Expectations are built during initial assessment while patient is placed in the shock position. The differential diagnosis is heat exhaustion. The rescuer tells her the following:

Mrs. Donnely, you can constrict or dilate your skin's blood vessels more or less when you need to. This means you can make them larger or smaller. This is a subconscious mechanism that you may not be aware of. It would be helpful, however, for you to imagine that your nervous system is directing just the right amount of dilation to help keep your body temperature at a safe level. Go ahead, now, and, in your own way, see or feel yourself responding positively to this need. Notice how your blood vessels are doing just exactly what they need to in order to keep you as cool and comfortable as is necessary.

Note that this directive does not use a metaphor like snow or cool water, although it would be fine to do so. Hypnotic suggestions for healing do not necessarily require the patient to have a detailed understanding of the specific medical condition or processes involved. The goal of hypnotic suggestion is to access the patient's subconscious mind, where beliefs and behaviors are formed, and make positive changes to those beliefs and behaviors. This can be done through general language and imagery that the patient can understand and relate to, rather than through technical or medical terminology. The patient should be able to understand the intent of the hypnotic suggestion, but not necessarily have a detailed understanding of the specifics of the condition or process being addressed. Whether or not you use such a direct suggestion or use a more descriptive metaphor depends on which one you believe will work best for the particular patient.

> *Situation: A man whose car ran out of gas attempted to walk along the desert freeway to find a gasoline station. After several hours of walking, he collapsed on the side of the road. A passerby stops, notes that the man's skin is very hot, dry, and flushed. He parks the car so as to place the man in the shade, then flags down another vehicle that goes for help. Neither car has water available. The passerby speaks to the man.*

Listen to me. Help is on the way. For now, it is very important that you become as cool as possible. You can do this now by doing exactly what I say. Will you do what I say? [Patient indicates that he will.] Good. Now, when I count to three, I want you to see yourself, in your mind's eye, plunging into a very cold lake. You are wearing a life preserver, and there is nothing for you to do but to enjoy the cold, comfortable, refreshing sensation of the water. One, two, three. Now, feel and see yourself plunging into that cold lake. Notice how your body temperature is already beginning to lower. Good. Now, maintain that temperature and that feeling while we wait for the ambulance. Good.

Cold Exposure

Hypothermia is also a danger when temperature mechanisms react to extreme environmental conditions in this case, cold. The rate and amount of heat loss by the body can be modified through a variety of metabolic systems that are controlled by the nervous system and that can be triggered by directives. Ski patrol rescuers have reported finding patients who survived a night on cold mountain trails without proper protection. In some cases, patients stated that they were able to stay warm by *imagining* that they were in a warm place. There are also scientific studies showing that hypnosis can modify thermoregulatory responses to cold.[7]

Exercise

You arrive at the emergency scene and find a ten-year-old child who has been scalded by hot water. Write what you would say to the child, using a strategy for gaining rapport, a strategy for building positive expectations, and appropriate guidelines for an effective directive.

Notes

1 Patterson, D.R., Goldberg, M.L., & Ehde, D.M. (September, 2011). Hypnosis in the treatment of patients with severe burns. *American Journal of Clinical Hypnosis*, 38(3), 200–212, DOI: 10.1080/00029157.1996.10403338
2 Wiechman, S.A., Patterson, D.R., Jensen, M.P., & Sharar, S.R. (August, 2007). A randomized controlled trial of hypnosis for burn wound care. *Rehabilitation Psychology*, 52(3), 247–253.
3 Omoigui, S. (August, 2007). The biochemical origin of pain: The origin of all pain is inflammation and the inflamatory response. Part 2 of 3- Inflammatory profile of pain syndromes. *Medical Hypotheses*, 69(6), 1169–1178.
4 Mawdsley, J.E. (2008). Hypnosis reduces measures of inflammation in patients with active ulcerative colitis. *Nature Reviews Gastroenterology & Hepatology*, 5(479). https://doi.org/10.1038/ncpgasthep1217
5 Time Magazine. (February, 1955). https://content.time.com/time/subscriber/article/0,33009,823748,00.html
6 Don Trent Jacobs YouTube presentation: https://www.youtube.com/watch?v=iVIMoE9scOA
7 Kissen, A.T., Reifler, C.B., & Thaler, V.H. (1964). Modification of thermoregulatory responses to cold by hypnosis. *Journal of Applied Physiology*, 19(6), 1043–1050. https://apps.dtic.mil/sti/pdfs/AD0613807.pdf

14 Respiratory Diseases

This chapter addresses communication approaches for the first responder responding to a situation where someone is having serious problems breathing.

Breath is life. It is no wonder patients suffering from acute respiratory disorders experience fear and panic. Beyond the cause of respiratory distress, such emotions themselves can negatively affect breathing patterns.[1] For example, hyperventilation associated with emotional states is relatively common. The person with labored breathing thus creates a vicious cycle, spiraling ever downward. With proper communication strategies, this cycle can be broken.[2] Furthermore, the initial bronchospasm characteristics of many respiratory problems can effectively be controlled with suitably presented directives.

Trauma, asthma, hyperventilation, pneumonia, choking, allergic reaction … there is a long list of reasons a patient may have difficulty breathing. When evaluating the airway, it is important not to make assumptions without a full physical assessment and all available diagnostics including pulse oximetry. As we have discussed, the first responder is communicating with the patient who is hyper-suggestible, owing to the natural hypnotic state that can be assumed during the first hour of trauma. Words that can calm and reassure can be life-saving.

I had a patient who I saw walk himself into the emergency department with a "fear of doom" look about him while grasping his throat as if he was choking. He was high anxiety and confused from lack of oxygen. The nurse confidently and positively handled the situation by motivating the patient to lie down in bed and slow down his breathing. When he became combative, the nurse still did not administer oxygen and tried to hold him down in an effort to protect the patient. The patient stopped breathing and was intubated. Later it was discovered that the patient had neck trauma and recovered after surgery. I am convinced that this patient would have benefited from a nurse who confidently gives reassurance, oxygen, and allowed him to sit up versus holding him down.

If a patient is having an airway emergency, it is important that you are following the correct path for that patient depending on the situation. Some patients need to sit up to breathe better, other patients may do better on their side in the recovery position. All patients with breathing problems require emergency

DOI: 10.4324/9781003430261-17

care with advanced life support diagnostics. Sometimes lethal issues like heart problems or sepsis can first present as difficulty breathing.

I have had patients stop breathing completely. When this type of deterioration occurs, it is important to remember the different audiences you have listening. The patient is still listening, the family members might be there, and of course your teammates. All of the people involved in the situation are susceptible to the way you respond. If you come across as scared or frantic, then everyone else can end up with that same energy especially because it comes from the leader.

Asthma

When a person has an asthma attack, a life-threatening emergency exists in that person's mind. The inability to take a normal breath evokes fear and fear, in return, induces a full asthma attack.[3] The patient's entire attention is concentrated on the next breath. For this reason, it is often difficult for the rescuer to get the patient's attention sufficiently to gain rapport and give appropriate directives. One suggestion is the use of a joining-in strategy.

Situation: A thirty-six-year-old housewife is in the throes of an asthma attack when the rescuer arrives at the woman's home. She is sitting on a kitchen chair, desperately gripping the chair's arms while she struggles for each breath. The rescuer approaches the patient so that their face is near the face of the patient. The rescuer then begins to mimic the labored breathing rate of the patient while talking.

June, listen ... to ... me. It's really ... hard to get... a breath, ... isn't it? And ... I know ... how frightening that can be. But notice ... just notice ... that it is beginning to get ... a bit easier now.

At this point, the rescuer's breathing begins to sound less labored. In many cases, the patient's own breathing rate will begin to keep pace with the rescuer's. As the breathing rates become slower, the rescuer acknowledges the improvement with comments such as "Good," "That's fine," and so on.

June, I have some pure, fresh oxygen for you that will help even more. As you inhale the oxygen, notice how much more relaxed your bronchiole's become when you exhale."[When giving the oxygen, the rescuer avoids placing the mask directly on the patient's face, as this might increase the anxiety.]

The standard treatment to be given by prehospital care personnel includes the administration of oxygen. If oxygen is available, the joining-in strategy can be used while it is being set up. In many instances, the patient will regain normal breathing even before the oxygen is administered. In any event, to enhance the benefit of the oxygen and to prevent further anxiety resulting from administering the oxygen, proper communication is also important. Once the rescuer gets the patient's attention and has gained a positive rapport with the joining-in strategy, a specific directive to relax the muscles around the bronchi upon exhalation can be given to the asthma patient if the dyspnea continues.

Research at the Walter Reed Hospital in Washington, D.C., has shown that such specific directives have actual physiological effects on the bronchial tubes. In the research, participants inhaled a chemical that brings on an asthma attack. Measurements of forced exhalation were taken with and without directives. Directives given to participants during hypnotic states of consciousness resulted in significant increases in exhalation volume, revealing that the directives had a direct physiological influence on the bronchioles that were in spasm. Now, returning to our example, we can continue our efforts to help June deal with an asthma attack using words that help with visualization and relaxation:

June, your breathing … is … becoming a little … easier now because you are beginning to *let* the muscles around your bronchi relax as you exhale. Just *continue* … to *allow* … those muscles to relax. That's good. You know, most people think that when you wheeze you can't get air into the lungs, but you and I know differently. We know it's just the opposite. When you are having an attack, you can't get the air out of the lungs to let fresh air in *until* you allow the bronchi muscles to relax as you are doing now. Just like your hand would open if you held a hot potato instead of closing, when you breathe in the oxygen, your bronchioles open up when they are full of oxygen.

In addition, to relieve the asthma attack at the emergency scene, the rescuer has an opportunity to explain to the asthma sufferer that they have the ability to "turn off" their wheezing anytime they need to. It can be explained that anyone suffering from asthma has simply developed a sensitivity to some irritant, possibly including biochemicals produced during emotional stress. The result is a learned response that triggers a complex of processes that cause mucus production and bronchospasm. Just as the nervous system has learned to respond to these sensitivities, it can also learn to stop the response, just as it did during the emergency call. In many cases, this comparatively simple and brief post-emergency dialogue will prevent severe asthma attacks from ever occurring again. This is especially true when the patient is a child.

Hyperventilation

Hyperventilating patients are also terrified of dying and have the feeling that it is impossible to get enough air into the lungs, in spite of the fact that they actually have breathed in too much oxygen. The immediate objective of the rescuer is to calm the patient and to raise the level of arterial carbon dioxide. Although this can be done effectively by having the patient rebreathe exhaled air from a paper bag, effective communication at the scene can also make a significant contribution to patient response and treatment outcome.

Situation: A twenty-four-year-old woman began hyperventilating after receiving news that her father had passed away. On arrival at the scene, the rescuer diagnoses that the patient is having a panic attack and the symptoms are a result of fast breathing.

Joan, slow your breathing down now. Exhale on my count only! One, two, three. That's better. Joan, I know how frightened you are, and how upset you must be, but you will feel better soon. Right now, you have inhaled too much oxygen, even though it seems like you aren't getting enough. By breathing into and out of this mask, you can balance out just the right amount of oxygen in your system and will feel better immediately. Go ahead and breathe into the mask and notice how much more relaxed you are beginning to feel.

Notice that, for this emergency patient, an authoritarian, commanding approach is appropriate at the outset, followed by a more compassionate, understanding statement. This is usually the best way to gain rapport and give directives to a person suffering a panic attack.

Choking

Many emergency situations arise when an airway is partially obstructed by some substance, such as a piece of meat. Since standard medical treatment is to avoid back blows or Heimlich maneuvers as long as the patient is able to exchange some air, communication is important for preventing respiratory distress from accelerating because of fear.

Situation: A forty-nine-year-old male has choked on a piece of meat in a restaurant. When the rescuer arrives on the scene, the patient is gasping desperately for breath, and people are gathered around him. While supporting the airway in its most efficient position, the rescuer projects confidence gains rapport and builds expectations before giving specific directives. The rescuer speaks slowly and calmly:

OK, Sir. I'm a paramedic, and you're going to be all right. It looks like you've got a piece of food started down the wrong pipe. I'm going to give you some pure oxygen [if available] that will help you feel better until we can get it out. In the meantime, I want you to do as I say. Will you do that? [Rescuer makes a direct contract.] Good. Now I want you just to continue as you are doing because right now you are getting enough oxygen. When we get you to the hospital the docs can remove the food easily, and you'll be good as new. I'm not going to try myself because I don't want to get it lodged to where it stops the exchange of air you are now able to achieve.

The patient is now prepared for the following directive:

Now, I want you to imagine that you are sipping your oxygen through a straw, getting just enough to enjoy the quality of the air and to sustain your vital systems. Remain in as comfortable a position as you choose, and sip, rather than try to gulp, that air slowly, savoring every drop. Good. Now, notice how efficiently your body is able to utilize such small quantities of oxygen. And, notice how much easier it is for you to breathe even now through the small opening yon air sipping your air through. Good.

Exercise

Using creative imagery of your own design, describe what you could say to a person with asthma that would help them visualize their breathing becoming more comfortable. After practicing with asthma, go on and practice how you would communicate with a patient hyperventilating or choking until the technique seems natural.

Notes

1 Whorwell, P.J., Houghton, L.A., Taylor, E.E., & Maxton, D.G. (July, 1992). Physiological effects of emotion: Assessment via hypnosis. *The Lancet*, 340, 69–72.
2 Anilo, H., Herer, B., Delignieres, A. et al (January, 2022). Hypnosis for the management of COPD-related anxiety and dysponoea in pulmonary rehabilitation. *National Library of Medicine*, 8, 1.
3 Cannizzaro, T. (December, 2019). Fear-induced Asthma. *Asthmanet.* https://asthma. net/living/fear-induced

15 Anaphylaxis

This chapter describes how words and thoughts can affect allergic reactivity in patients.

Anaphylaxis is a fairly common emergency that can be life-threatening. It occurs when someone has been sensitized to some substance at some point in time and then reacts violently to subsequent contact. Offending agents include drugs (especially penicillin), certain foods, medicines, chemicals, and the sting of an insect. In essence, the cause of an anaphylactic reaction is a hypersensitive immune system response to some foreign substance. The system somehow learned to be overprotective in defending the body against future invasions from a one-time intruder. The immune system releases its own chemicals that cause someone to go into shock—a rapid decrease in blood pressure and inability to breathe. Exactly why the mind–body complex chooses to develop antibodies for a specific substance more aggressively than for another is not known. Emotional factors, however, at the time of the initial exposure, may be involved. In 2004, more than 300 empirical articles were analyzed describing a significant relationship between psychological stress and the suppression of immune function.[1]

Advanced-level treatment for anaphylaxis includes the use of oxygen and drugs like epinephrine, Benadryl, and steroids that a paramedic would normally carry in an advanced-level ambulance. All cases of anaphylaxis require an emergency call for this level of care because of the risk of deterioration. Position yourself to use hypnotic communication during moments when you can be reassuring. For example, while waiting on the ambulance to arrive—be reassuring with the use of visualization. Also, when the paramedic is administering drugs—be reassuring with expectations.

Redirecting the Patient's Immune System

Directives given by a confident rescuer to a frightened emergency patient (who can be considered to be in a hypnotic state of consciousness) influence messages to and from the autonomic nervous system. The communication objective of

DOI: 10.4324/9781003430261-18

the rescuer responding to an anaphylactic reaction emergency is to redirect the overreaction of the immune system to the specific antigen. In addition to giving directives that can reverse bronchospasm, the other following signs of anaphylaxis can be targeted:

1   Inflammation and itching of the skin (hives)
2   Inflammation and edema in the larynx
3   Dilation of blood vessels and capillaries (reducing the amount of fluid in the vessels)
4   Continual release of the chemical, histamine, that causes the above condition.

Memory in the Immune System

Immunological memory continues long after an original infection.[2] This helps the immune system more effectively deal with pathogens previously encountered. As has been stated, the anaphylactic reaction results from a previously learned association with some substance or antigen. Sometimes the antigen itself is relatively harmless, but the body will attack the substance. Sometimes a memory of the original event can trigger an unnecessary immune reaction. Since memory implies images, even if at the cellular level, then we can begin to understand why words that form images might influence memory responses. New cellular "programs" can be imagined that replace older ones.

A fascinating and still controversial example of this was published in the June 1988 issue of the prestigious British journal, *Nature*.[3] A French immunologist, Jacques Benveniste, took a common antibody (IgE) and exposed it to certain white cells in the blood called *basophils*. When this is done, the IgE typically attaches itself to certain receptor sites on the cells and waits to attack an antigen. The experiment began when Dr. Benveniste mixed the blood serum containing the white cells and IgE with a solution prepared from goat's blood that contained an anti-IgE (antigen). Dr. Benveniste knew that this would cause the antibody (IgE) to set off an allergic response resulting in the release of histamine. Then Benveniste diluted the anti-IgE goat blood mixture tenfold and added it again to the human blood. The same reaction occurred. He kept on diluting, time after time, until the anti-IgE solution was diluted so drastically that it contained one part antibody to 10^{120} parts water. Mathematically, at this point, it was impossible for the water to contain a single molecule of antibody. The solution, however, which was basically now just distilled water, continued to set off the histamine reaction!

The experiment was positively duplicated many times by Benveniste and by researchers in Israel, Canada, and Italy. Still yet, other scientists scoffed at his conclusions, and it remains controversial even now long after Benveniste's death.[4] We share it here as at least a possible rationale for emergency hypnosis being an effective adjunct to standard care in potentially saving someone's life who is in anaphylactic shock, one also supported by anecdotal events. For example, author Four Arrows used self-hypnosis to save his life after anaphylactic shock stopped his breathing. Also, in his book, *Quantum Healing*, Dr. Deepak Chopra, relates an anecdotal story that supports Benveniste's theory. His father, a cardiologist in India, was once stationed as an army doctor in Jammu. His mother suffered there from severe asthma and anaphylactic reactions to the pollen of a native flower that blossomed every spring. To avoid this, every spring his father drove his mother to Kashmir, where the air was free of this particular pollen and where she was delighted by the beauty of the mountain valley.

One spring the heavy rains had made the road impassable for the return trip to Jammu, so they chartered an airplane and returned home early. When the plane landed, the mother's skin began to welt and blister, and she had difficulty breathing. When the steward ran up to her, the father said, "There's nothing you can do. It's the pollen in Jammu." The steward looked puzzled and explained that they had not yet landed in Jammu, but at Udhampur, their first stop. Within moments, Chopra's mother stopped struggling for breath, and her sores vanished on the spot.

Situation: A twenty-two-year-old female, allergic to bee stings, was stung in the neck while gardening. She immediately called the fire department. Within minutes the fire department arrives on the scene and finds the patient with swelling about the lips and tongue, red and itching skin, and stomach cramps. The patient is anxious and complains that the reaction is going to get much worse. After accomplishing the credibility, rapport, and expectation objectives indicated by the first three letters of the CREDIBLE mnemonic (while the stinger is removed and oxygen is administered), the following directive is given by the rescuer while waiting for the paramedics.

Sally, I want you to listen to me carefully now. Have you ever gotten goose pimples on your skin after thinking about something exciting or scary? Did they stay and get worse, or did they go away when you stopped thinking about them? *[Patient responds that they went away.]*

Your reaction to the bee sting is similar to the goose bump reaction. The stinger is out and the substance has dissipated into your bloodstream. Your body has forgotten how to turn off the reaction. But you can do that now. I just want you to imagine that those antibodies that keep producing the chemicals making your skin red and swollen have been called off. They have been thanked for trying their best to attack the bee venom but were told that they were much more aggressive than they needed to be. And, now that the venom has been dissipated in your blood stream, they can stop and allow your body to return to a cool and comfortable state.

Just begin to feel your blood vessels constricting again and see in your mind's eye all the chemical processes that started a few minutes ago beginning to reverse. Notice that your throat and face are beginning to feel cooler and more comfortable already.

Although poison oak or ivy reactions do not often constitute an emergency crisis, they occasionally do. Even less serious cases can cause a great deal of suffering. In his 1968 book, *Clinical Hypnotherapy*, Dr. David Cheek states in the concluding remarks of his chapter "Emergency Uses and Spontaneous Trance,"

> Emergency uses of hypnosis are numerous and the valuable possibilities obvious with such urgent situations as highway accidents, burns, cardiac arrest, surgical shock, status asthmaticus, and any crisis where a patient seems to have lost motivation toward recovery. We have not explored all the ways in which a body can cope with cancer, with acute dermatitis like poison oak.

One day when Four Arrows returned from a putting out a wildfire when he worked for Marin County Fire Department, one of the volunteer helpers came to him and expressed apprehension about having breathed in smoke from poison oak. He appeared desperate as he told me that he had almost died owing to it causing anaphylactic shock. He felt sure that handling the hose that was pulled through the bushes and breathing in the smoke would result in a catastrophic and disabling reaction. With a sound of matter-of-factness in my voice, I assured him that the response to poison oak was an autonomic nervous system activity that could easily be modified with a new inner belief system. He was frightened enough to be hyper-suggestible to what I was saying, and it was therefore unnecessary to hypnotize him formally. I asked him to get comfortable in a chair and to tell his body that *this* time he would only experience a mild rash. I told him that he would be able to see the rash, but that it would be so comfortable he would not feel it. The next morning he came to me overjoyed. A mild red rash appeared on his arms, belly, and neck. He claimed that there was no itching. This was quite a difference from the anaphylactic shock.

Exercise

You have a patient allergic to bee sting who has been stung on the foot by a yellow jacket. Ten minutes have elapsed, and the swelling is increasing steadily. You are with the patient during transport to the hospital. Practice talking to someone real or to an imagined person in this situation who is going into anaphylactic shock. If you can record yourself. Practicing will help you gain confidence in best ways to go through our Mnemonic, CREDIBLE.

Notes

1 Segerstrom, S.C., & Miller, G.E. (July, 2004). Psychological stress and the human immune system: A meta-analytic study of 30 years of inquiry. *Psychological Bulletin,* 130(4), 601–630. https://www.ncbi.nlm.nih.gov/pmc/articles/PMC1361287/
2 Janeway, C.A. Jr., Travers, P. et al. (2001). *Immunobiology: The Immune System in Health and Disease.* 5th edition. Garland Science.
3 Benveniste, J. (2004). *The British Medical Journal.* https://www.bmj.com/content/329/7477/1290
4 Pincock, S. (November, 2004). Jacques Benveniste. *The Lancet.* https://www.thelancet.com/journals/lancet/article/PIIS0140-6736(04)17339-X/fulltext

16 Childbirth and Pediatric Emergencies

This chapter illustrates communication strategies relating to emergency childbirth situations, defining an emergency as when a birth is about to happen in an unexpected place or at an unexpected time that instigates a call for help. The chapter also discusses the potential for hypnotic communication when working with young children.

Childbirth Emergencies

Professional first responders are usually trained in the basics related to assisting with child birth, including:

- Determining frequency of contractions
- Asking about prenatal history
- Checking blood pressure and checking for vaginal bleeding
- Looking for positioning of baby
- Assuring oxygen is sufficient
- Attention to umbilical cord
- Evaluate for crowning.

If any of these problems exist, then using the directives in previous chapters relating to blood pressure, pain, bleeding, etc., can be used. If there seem to be no complications and the mother is confident, nature can take its course with little need for hypnotic directives beyond encouragement and confidence building. However, many women, especially young and unprepared mothers-to-be, may be significantly stressed by pain, or lack of the medical assistance they may have intended. Pain, hemorrhage, toxemia, and even infection might relate to undue stress and fear during labor.

Although some levels of anxiety is considered normal during labor, excessive anxiety is an emotional factor that results in severe pain due to a decrease in

DOI: 10.4324/9781003430261-19

pelvic blood flow and increased muscle tension, as a result of an increasè in the secretion of catecholamines.[1]

Here is where the hypnotic language comes into play. As someone responding to a childbirth situation, your priority is to project confidence, establish a positive rapport, and build positive expectations with the mother. Any of the strategies presented in the earlier chapters can be used to accomplish these three objectives. Subsequent directives used to enhance a positive delivery should continue to dispel worries and fears.

Situation: A twenty-four-year-old woman is in her first stage of labor. The amniotic sac ruptured moments after the rescuer arrived on the scene. The ambulance service is too far away, so the family station wagon is used to transport the mother to the hospital, which is thirty minutes away. This will be the woman's second pregnancy; her first child was aborted at six months. The rescuer has attained good rapport with the mother, and sterile supplies for delivery are ready in case the birth happens before reaching the hospital. The rescuer gives her positive reassurances:

Mary, soon your child will be born and will see you from the outside for the first time. From now on your only focus is the amazing experience of birthing, regardless of whatever labor is needed. You are going to have your baby with a great big smile on your face, whether before or after we get to the hospital. At any point along the way you might become temporarily distracted from your *positive focus because of your labor and the work you two are doing for the birth.* That's quite all right, because as soon as I say, "focus," you will return to focus on that comfortable effort that we call labor. You can do this because the only thing that is really on your mind is the fact that, in a little while, you will be seeing the wonderful baby you've been waiting for. There is nothing to bother. Nothing that can interfere with your having your baby as quickly and easily as possible.

In many cases, the woman involved in an emergency childbirth will have a relatively optimistic attitude on her own. The above directives serve to maintain this optimism throughout the many worries and annoyances that might occur during the labor. In some cases, however, the woman will enter labor without this optimism. Instead, worry, fear, and even guilt are dominant emotions. Women who are unhappy with their pregnancy and/or are afraid of the pain and possible complication they *believe* to be probable can create some of the problems listed earlier. Although the above directive may suffice to alleviate such concerns, a more direct approach may be more effective *if* you know in advance just what those concerns are.

To find out what these fears are, you could simply ask the woman, "Do you have any worries, concerns, or fears about your delivery?" However, according to the late David Cheek, a well-known hypnotherapist and a diplomate of the American Board of Obstetrics and Gynecology who pioneered much of the research that associates psychological states during pregnancy and labor with a variety of physical and mental responses, such a question may be contraindicated. He once said that asking such a question might cause the person to think of fears that otherwise would not have come into her mind. According to Dr. Cheek, the best way to find out if a pregnant woman has a sufficiently healthy attitude about giving birth is with ideomotor responses. He suggests asking a neutral question like "Do you know or have a guess as to whether you are going to have a boy or a girl?" If the woman commits herself to a decision, his research shows that it is likely that the attitude is positive. A "yes or no" response is generally an indication that there are not fears. If the response indicates, I don't know, or I don't want to answer, then there may be some significant apprehension.

Setting up the ideomotor response[2] is an easy thing to do with the woman in labor. Here is an example:

Mary, I want you to go ahead and concentrate on those deep, relaxing breaths. In the meantime, I want to ask you a few questions using a technique that won't interrupt your concentration. The only answers you need to give me are yes, no, or I don't know, which can also mean, I don't want to answer. Allow your unconscious mind to lightly raise your index finger [indicate which hand] for yes, your second finger for no, and your thumb for I don't know, or I don't want to answer. If you understand, let me know by raising the correct finger. Good.

At this point, the rescuer can ask some simple history questions or other questions that can easily lead into the opportunity to ask about the baby's sex or other simple questions.

- Is this your first pregnancy?
- Does the moist towel on your forehead still feel cool?
- Is someone going to meet you at the hospital?

If the thumb raises, this indicates an unwillingness to make a commitment to making a decision that is likely rooted in some kind of apprehension. The source of possible fears is often in material, television, or conversations with well-meaning friends and relatives that have produced images about giving birth being an ordeal. There might also be financial concerns, relationship problems, and so on. In any event, if the thumb responds, you can then continue with more direct interrogations about a potential fear by asking more directly, "Are there any worries, fears, or concerns that are troubling you now?" If the response is "no," just accept the answer and continue with the directives presented earlier. If the response is either "yes," or "I don't know," then it is usually quite easy to expose the problem and resolve the fear with a few reassuring sentences that help dilute the concern. Once accomplished, return to the original directive and repeat it.

Pediatric Emergencies

The first responder attending a child suffering from a medical emergency has a special opportunity. Not only can their actions and words help save the child from a permanent, disabling injury, but also they can significantly influence the child's response to future injuries or illnesses, as well as to future interventions by medical personnel. Furthermore, of all age groups, children generally have the greatest capacity for visual imagery to have a hypnotic influence. Once a positive rapport with a child is attained, little to no preparation is necessary to go right into what might be considered dramatic directives.

Because of this extreme suggestibility to words and the images they create, it is especially important to monitor or prevent well-intended but potentially damaging remarks from concerned relatives. If such remarks are heard by the child, simply rephrasing them so the child can interpret them positively can reverse the negative effects quickly. This also serves to educate the parent to leave the communication to you. When establishing rapport with a child, it is important to remember that a stranger, even a uniformed one, alone may be frightening. (Note, in some cultures or communities the uniform can itself create mistrust or fear.) In any event, establishing a positive rapport is usually easy when the joining-in strategy is used at the outset.

The joining-in strategy works so well to get children and adolescents into your confidence because most adults tend to alienate them with their language. Children will respond best when what they hear from an adult is an acknowledgment of what he or she is really feeling and thinking. For example, "Wow, I bet it's scary being out here with all these people standing around, huh?" might help a first responder gain immediate rapport.

Using a situation we previously used to stop bleeding is a good example for joining-in with a child:

Situation: A three-year-old female was left unattended for a few minutes. She walked to a kennel that contained six huskies bred for sled racing. One of the dogs knocked her down and the others jumped on her, biting and pawing at her (apparently in play). Her father heard her screams and rescued her from the dogs after several minutes. By then she had suffered a lacerated cornea, a ripped ear, several puncture wounds on her legs, arms, and face, and a large avulsion on the back of her hand. The fire department was called and arrives within minutes. The little girl is screaming hysterically at that time. Upon approach, the rescuer lifts the child's hand and looks directly and only at the avulsion—this helps narrow the focus of the little girl to just one thing at the outset:

Oh, boy, I'll bet that hand really hurts. And look at how your skin is folded back like that. I'll bet you didn't know what your skin looked like underneath before. Well, do you know that that will feel more comfortable if you fold the skin back to where it was? [At this point the child is still crying, but she has paid enough attention to become interested in what the firefighter is talking about.]

Why don't you go ahead and fold that skin back; then you can help me take care of your other sores. OK. Here, just use this sterile cloth and put the skin right back where it was. (He places the 4-by-4-inch bandage in her other hand.) Good, now just lift right here and lay the skin flap right back down again. (The child stops crying and follows the instructions.)

From this point on, the child participates in treating all of the wounds that she can reach. Each one is talked about as though it is a special, important item. To keep the emphasis on the child remaining relatively painfree, a game is set up whereby the paramedic claims he can find the wound that "feels the best." When a more hurtful wound is discussed, it is quickly treated and the search for the "best" wound continues. By this time, less than five minutes from the start, the child is smiling and conversing freely. Once the wounds are superficially treated, the rescuer begins discussing the dogs.

You know, I'll bet those dogs really feel sad about what they did. They are used to playing rough like that with each other. They just didn't know how to play with a little girl. I'll bet when you get your own dogs you can teach them how to play with you, can't you? [Response is positive.] Good. And, I'll bet you could even teach them how to play with little boys and girls if you are older when you get a dog.

With this simple communication, the likely chance of the child having a phobia about dogs in later years is probably reduced. When the ambulance arrives, the rescuer should introduce the child to the paramedics and explain exactly what happened. Giving her praise for how she handled the situation will strengthen her even more.

Situation: A twelve-year-old boy was badly beaten by his father. When the father left the house, neighbors brought the child to the fire station. The child appeared to be suffering significant pain in numerous locations. After the confidence, rapport, and expectation aspects of the CREDIBLE mnemonic are handled effectively, and the appropriate medical treatments are being administered, along with possibly having someone privately contact the police to report the incident, the following directives for pain control were given.

Louis, I want you to close your eyes for a little while because I'm going to show you how to do something that will make you feel more comfortable. Now, as you close your eyes, you can let your whole body just go limp, just the way a wet towel does when you drop it on the floor.

This particular directive serves to assure that the child is in that state of consciousness that will indeed make him highly receptive to the pain control directives that will follow. This is done because of the time that elapsed between the actual beating and the visit to the fire station. Although the child is still frightened, the possibility that spontaneous hyper-suggestibility may have relinquished itself to left-brain thinking is there. Since children can quickly be brought back into this receptive state of consciousness with simple requests to imagine relaxing feelings, such a directive can always be used before more specific ones are given.

Good. Now I want you to imagine a long row of light switches. Above each switch is a colored bulb, all turned on, and each one a different color. There's a blue one and a yellow one and a green one. What other colors do you see? (The child answers "yellow and red.") Good.

Now, these switches all have round knobs on them that allow you to turn down the light and make it dimmer. Or, you can turn it down all the way until the light is off. This light system is very much like your own nervous system. It sends messages to and from your brain to all the parts of your body. And it can turn down or turn off different feelings in the body. Now, let me show you how this works. (At this point, the rescuer assigns one of the light switches to an *uninjured* part of the body. In this case, it is the child's left hand.) Imagine that your hand is connected to the blue light switch. Now start turning down the dimmer until the light is almost off. Notice that your hand is beginning to become like wood. I can pinch it and you won't hardly feel it. (Medic pinches the skin between the finger and thumb and asks the child it hurt. When the child indicates it did not, which is usually what happens, then say): Now, turn the blue light back on so you have normal feeling in that hand, and let's assign some light switches to places on your body where you would like to feel more comfortable.

This technique allowed the child to turn down or turn off his pain anywhere he chooses very quickly. As for the emotional pain that is likely related to having been hurt by his father, this would be dealt with hopefully by qualified people down the line.

True or False

1 Women about to give birth seldom have any fear or anxieties that can make the event difficult.
2 Children involved in a medical emergency are not as receptive to suggestions as are adults.
3 The joining-in strategy is very effective with children.
4 The effectiveness of emergency treatment of young children can affect their reactions to future trauma.

Notes

1 Lowe, N.K. (1996). The pain and discomfort of labor and birth. *Journal of Obstetric, Gynecologic & Neonatal Nursing*, 25(1), 82–92.
2 Shenefelt, P.D. (2011). Ideomotor signaling: From divining spiritual messages to discerning subconscious answers during hypnosis and hypnoanalysis, a historical perspective. *American Journal of Clinical Hypnosis*, 53, 157–167.

17 Psychological Emergencies

First responders often are called to situations where a psychological crisis not involving a physical injury or illness is occurring putting the victim and possibly others in danger of physical harm. This chapter discusses several examples and offers effective communication strategies for each.

Although many emergency patients experience psychological crises as a component of their physical injury or illness, this chapter is devoted to those cases where the emotional status alone is the basis for risk. Some examples of psychological emergencies include sudden depression, suicide attempts or threats, rape, sexual assault, behavior threatening harm to others, or acute psychosis or hallucinations. Although gaining rapport with a patient is always crucial for effective directives, it is especially paramount when working with a psychologically disturbed individual. This is especially challenging to the rescuer since, in these emergencies, patients have a limited potential for overt response. It is therefore more difficult to know when rapport has actually been achieved. With continual communication efforts using the CREDIBLE mnemonic, a rescuer has a better chance to help the patient regain control of their thinking and behaviors. Below we offer a few examples of situations first responders are likely to encounter.

Death of a Loved One Emergencies

Each person responds so uniquely to the death of a loved one, and each situation is so different that it is difficult to list general communication strategies. The following guidelines and case studies, however, do describe some consistently effective tactics.

First, the rescuer should realize that some type of emotional or physical response is a normal part of the grief process. Respect the grieving person's need for sympathy and follow their wishes if they seem relatively harmless. Allow a hysterical individual to do what they want, however, can be a difficult call. For example, is it best to let a hysterical woman continue to hold on to her husband who just died from a gunshot wound? What if it was a badly injured child?

DOI: 10.4324/9781003430261-20

In any case, it is important to be truthful and direct with the surviving person, whom we will refer to as the "patient." They will likely be hyper-intuitive and focused on the facts, and indirect statements or partial truths will often disrupt rapport and trust. If the patient screams demanding to know if someone they discovered in the bathroom with slit wrists is "really dead?" and you know the person is, it is generally better to tell the truth. Exceptions to this rule might include a situation where the news could significantly aggravate a medical condition in the living patient.

Joining in strategies with the patient can be effective. By doing this, the rescuer and the patient enter into a bond. In the following case, the rescuer joins in and encourages the patient's overwhelming grief, then gradually directs them in ways that can calm them. It is important to allow for or encourage actual crying. Crying serves as a catharsis for pain and tension. With crying, blood pressure at first goes up, but then it tends to lower afterward. It also allows for more efficient breathing because crying activates the parasympathetic nervous system, slowing breathing and heart rate.[1] "Researchers have established that crying releases oxytocin and endogenous opioids, also known as endorphins. These feel-good chemicals help ease both physical and emotional pain."[2]

> *Situation: A thirty-four-year-old woman and her seven-year-old son crashed their car into the side of a cliff on a winding road trying to avoid a deer. The car burst into flames on impact. The woman escaped unharmed, but could not reach through the flames to get her son out of the car. Several people passing by stopped to help. One person restrained the woman from going near the burning car while the other tried his best to open the door. By the time the fire department arrives, the boy is severely burned and obviously dead. The mother is hysterical and is calling for her boy. Several times she screams, "My God, he's burned to death!" The rescuer approaches the woman calmly and professionally, then firmly takes her by the arm and walks her two steps away from the crowd:*

Ma'am, it's time to cry. Your son has passed away, and there's nothing we can do for him now but to cry for his loss and allow your mourning and your loving feelings help send off his spirit. Let the other firemen do their job. I'll stay with you and help you. The worst is over now.

Throughout this communication, the rescuer provides sincere support for the woman by joining in with her grief. Sharing of the sadness in this way adds to the effectiveness of the joining-in strategy. The shared grieving causes the pain and suffering of the moment to diminish enough for her to regain control. As she begins to respond to the rescuer's questions, she also becomes ready to listen to directives that will lead her into the ambulance and away from the scene. In many instances, relatives at the scene of an emergency suffer from psychological crisis at the onset of a medical crisis with a loved one, when death is feared but has not yet occurred. While first responders work on the medical patient, this person's behavior can be damaging to themself and to the primary patient who has become suddenly ill or injured. Joining in with this person's feelings and then gradually taking control of the feelings is again very effective. Simply acknowledging the distraught person's feelings can have a noticeable calming effect. Thus, instead of saying, "It's OK, he's going to be fine; just calm down," say, "You're real scared, but we are going to take good care of him."

This simple statement tends to build instant rapport. Once this is accomplished, a directive should be given that is meaningful to the person and that should partially distract them from the emotional trauma. For example, you can say, "I need you to help me take care of your husband. I need you to calm down, go to that corner, and wait for the ambulance."

Suicide Attempt

When evaluating a patient who is suspected of depression or suicidal thoughts it is important to get them to communicate. You are trying to evaluate them to see if they are a danger to themselves or someone else. Some patients may have already tried to kill themselves while others have a plan to do so. The patient must trust you enough to allow you to figure out what has transpired or might transpire. Some people, especially if they have a healthcare background, may be difficult to get an honest story because they want to avoid going to a psych hospital. So, it is important to look at the environment and also interview others around your patient.

It is okay to ask blunt questions in a caring way:

"Are you feeling especially negative about things in your life right now?"
"Have you been thinking about suicide now or in the past?"
"How are you able to deal with your life stress right now?"
"Do you have any plans for how you might kill yourself to make it all go away?"

Look for signs that show your patient has a disregard for safety as if they do not care about their life. One time I arrived in my ambulance at a car that hit a sign in a ditch. I figured out that the patient had no brake marks on the pavement and that led me to uncover the source of the wreck was not an accident, it was a suicide attempt. Other concerning signs to look for include a patient who gets their affairs in order with no logical reasoning or a patient who makes matter-of-fact statements like, "I wish I were dead." These behaviors should be taken seriously and deeply questioned even if made in a joking manner.

In the following case, the grieving wife of a man who died from a cocaine overdose attempted suicide while the medics were still on the scene. Although the man was dead, CPR efforts were initiated and could not be stopped (legally) until the paramedic team reached the hospital and the man was pronounced dead by a physician.

> *Situation: One fire fighter remains in the area and returns to the house to check on the wife and obtain information for his report. He walks into the house and finds the woman collapsed on the floor. An empty bottle of pheno-barbital pills lays at her side. Her respirations are failing, and her pulse rate is falling. After calling for another ambulance and mutual aid from another fire department, the fire fighter begins giving strategic directives to the unconscious woman while administering oxygen:*

Mrs. Davis, listen to me. The worst is over now. Whatever has happened to your husband, there is still much for you to do. If you had any guilt about anything, that guilt is now leaving you. If you have any anger, that anger is leaving as well. Now you are going to be reborn into life for yourself. With each breath that passes through your lungs, your body will cleanse out the chemicals you took to gain relief from your grief. As these chemicals clear out, you will feel your health returning. Soon you will begin to feel a lightness inside yourself as you move along your rebirth and return to life. Let every part of your body respond to this lightness, or is it a brightness? With each breath passing through your lungs, feel the chemicals being cleansed out of your body. Notice the new feeling of harmony with friends and family. Let that bright lightness carry you into your rebirth and return to life.

The fire fighter repeats this rhetoric for almost forty-five minutes, the time it takes for the next group of rescuers to arrive.

Rape Victim

In the emergency pre-hospital environment, it is not your job to learn about all of the details of the rape. The focus of your interaction should be centered on taking care of life-threatening injuries, preserving evidence, and comforting the patient with your words. The interview that uncovers the details of the event should be saved for law enforcement.

Victims of rape require significant emotional support that can be rapidly given with proper communication strategies. Whether the patient is withdrawn or hysterical, they should be treated with extreme gentleness and respect. Statements that reflect anger, disgust, or blame should be carefully avoided. The rescuer should not criticize the patient with comments such as, "You really shouldn't have been walking in this area," and so on. All words that are spoken should emphasize the fact that the worst is over. In such cases, this phrase can be so effective in calming and reassuring the patient that it can be helpful to ask them to repeat it to themself over and over again. By evoking their participation, either by repeating words you ask them to speak or by assisting in any first aid that may be necessary, the patient regains a sense of control that they desperately need to reclaim.

> *Situation: An ambulance team is called to a foster home. A nine-year old boy had been sodomized. He was surrounded by a policeman and counselors from the home, sitting and staring without talking. He would not talk to anyone and the ambulance was called for fear the boy was going into shock.*

One of the medics slowly stepped up to the boy. Before taking his vital signs or touching him he reached asked if it was alright if he tied the boy's shoe which was unlaced. He did this as a way to achieve rapport. Although the boy said nothing, the medic pretended if he had said "yes" and said, "Good, I'll do that now. I'm going to put a blood pressure cuff on your arm now. Is that OK? Just let me know by blinking your eyes." The boy's eyes blinked. The medic touched his left arm and said "This arm is the one I want to put the blood pressure cuff on, okay?"

Once it was determined the boy was not at risk for shock, the medic said.

> I know what happened to you hurts you in many ways now, but I promise you will be fine. You are a strong young man things are going to be better for you in a short while. Would you like to go for a ride with us in the ambulance? You can sit up front with us as we take you to a place where they will check you out to make sure you are OK?

The two medics ask if he would like to lay in the wheeled stretcher instead, but the boy stood up and shook his head, implying he preferred to sit in the front seat of the ambulance. His healing had begun.

Disruptive, Dangerous Behavior

Occasionally a first responder will encounter an extremely disruptive individual whose behavior could harm themself or others, including the rescuer. The causes for such behavior are many. Alcohol and drug use are the most common. Certain physical and mental conditions, from concussions to diabetic shock also may be responsible. For some people, this kind of behavior is their reaction to stress. In any case, the first responder's safest treatment is with using CREDIBLE. Convey loving confidence, build rapport quickly, encourage positive expectations, offer a directive that will help conjure an appropriate image that is sufficiently believable, will be taken literally and don't be over-enthusiastic. Throughout the process, avoid expressing any of your own anger or fear. Do not be heard using terms like *crazy* or *drunk*. Maintain a body posture that is nonaggressive. Even though you may be concerned for your own safety, avoid any action or statement that will make you "part of the enemy" or a target for the patient's violence.

The rapport strategy of choice with this kind of emergency is *feedback*, followed by a variation of the joining-in strategy. Speaking calmly, slowly, and directly to the patient, the rescuer should pay careful attention to what is being said. If the patient is not speaking, a question can be asked to elicit some statement. Whatever the patient says, the rescuer should wait a few moments, then give feedback with the same information. Then, the statement should be repeated, this time sounding as though the idea, thought, or feeling were the rescuer's own. In many instances, the statements will be negatively oriented toward someone. Nonetheless, the rescuer should continue the feedback and joining-in the charade until a positive rapport is established with the patient. Then, subsequent directives can diffuse the violence and belligerence.

> *Situation: A thirty-two-year-old male left a bar with a revolver and began shooting in the air and threatening to kill someone named Fred. The man was obviously under the influence of alcohol. After he had used up all the bullets in the gun, he threw it on the ground and took a pocket knife out of his pocket. He then challenged anyone to take it out of his hands, while occasionally continuing to talk about putting an end to Fred. The man's behavior was borderline hysterical, and fits of crying were intermittent. Several of his friends had attempted to approach him, with no success, when an off-duty police officer, knowledgeable in effective communication strategies, steps several yards in front of the disruptive patient.*

Rescuer: What's your name?

Patient: None of your damned business!

Rescuer: It's hot out tonight. Listen, you probably think that it's none of my business what your name is. Right?

Patient: That's right. Who are you?

Rescuer: You know, it's none of my business who you are, and I don't even know what I am doing out here, and I don't know this person you call Fred. But whatever he did or you think he did to you to make you this upset, I'm here to help you make it right somehow, OK?

At this point, the rescuer will know they have gained a rapport with the patient if there is any positive change in the patient's body language, eyes, or words. Disruptive patients do not tend to remember the words or thoughts they speak from one moment to the next, yet the feeling behind the words remains. Feeding back information and joining in the agreement are thus effective tactics for "becoming friends" with the person, especially when the cause of disruption is alcohol or drug-related. After the rapport is gained and dialogue exists between the two, the officer asks the man to walk away from the crowd so they can talk more. In a short while, the patient is crying in the police officer's arms about how his wife left him for his friend Fred.

Exercise

An eighteen-year-old boy just wrecked his father's car. He does not seem to be injured and is standing outside the car kicking it and throwing things from inside out dangerously onto the street. He angrily threatens those around him. You are a paramedic in uniform and arrive at the scene. Develop a dialogue that might allow you to gain his confidence and give effective suggestions for different behavior.

Notes

1 Leamey, T. (June, 2022). Crying is an important way to communicate and process emotions. *CNET*. https://www.cnet.com/health/medical/the-benefits-of-crying-and-why-its-good-for-your-health/#:~:text=Crying%20activates%20your%20parasympathetic%20 nervous,rate%20and%20bringing%20you%20relief.
2 Newhouse, L. (March, 2021). Is crying good for you. *Harvard Health Blog*. https://www.health.harvard.edu/blog/is-crying-good-for-you-2021030122020#: ~:text=Researchers%20have%20established%20that%20crying,both%20physical% 20and%20emotional%20pain.

18 Self-hypnosis

Professionals engaged in medical emergency responses know, no matter how rewarding, it can be very stressful and wearing on body, mind, and spirit. Using self-hypnosis is vital for maintaining a positive perspective and a healthy life. This chapter briefly describes how to do it effectively.

Trance-based learning, including self-learning with specific intentions, was a natural part of human life for most of its nature-based existence and still is for traditional Indigenous cultures that have managed to hold on to the spiritual/ceremonial/self-autonomous ways of life. The concept of "hypnosis," of course, was not known. It was natural. It was observed in animals. If a human wanted to be more confident, more generous, a better hunter or basket maker, more in tune with helping the community, etc., he or she generally know that willful determination was insufficient. Trance work, whether meditation, visualization or specific ceremonies were daily events.

Today science confirms the value of self-hypnosis as a highly effective tool for stress management and the control of anxiety and managing stress. It can also be used to retrain the mind to react differently to stressors and develop more positive habits that promote greater control and resilience in the face of stress. This includes using it to reframe and let go of negative hypnotically induced beliefs that allow us to tolerate logical inconsistencies, no matter how harmful or unhelpful they may be. As with patient communication in the field, a deep trance is not necessary for guiding the mind to cope with a crisis. Since by now you have acquired a thorough understanding of naturalistic hypnosis and may have gained confidence in its use with others, you will be able to commit yourself to use it as a learning strategy.

The most traditional way to hypnotize yourself is to start by putting yourself in a comfortable position. It does not matter whether you are lying down or sitting up as long as you are comfortable. You need to say nothing aloud, merely think of your suggestions. Your eyes should be closed and relaxation enhanced if you take two or three deep breaths. Then think, Now I am going into the

DOI: 10.4324/9781003430261-21

hypnotic state of consciousness. This is your first suggestion. Slowly repeat this suggestion in your mind three times, and you will begin to slip into hypnosis. To achieve a slightly greater depth, simply say to yourself, I am going deeper, more and more relaxed. You may want to imagine yourself going down an escalator while you count backward from ten to zero, seeing yourself step down with each count. Picture yourself stepping off at the bottom when you reach zero and being ready to receive instructions.

The eye-role is another induction that can be used effectively for self-hypnosis. This involves looking as high as possible with the eyes while at the same time taking a deep breath and closing the eyelids. After a moment, allow the eyes to lower while exhaling and visualizing a falling leaf. When the leaf finally falls to the ground, assume that you are in sufficient hypnosis to receive suggestions. There are many techniques for self-hypnosis available on the Internet.

Although you should take for granted that you are entering hypnosis following these inductions (so as not to disrupt it with doubting or analytical thinking), it may be helpful to confirm the state with a simple suggestion for a finger levitation. After the induction, simply imagine a feeling of weightlessness in your index finger and see it lifting slightly upwards as though a helium balloon is tied to it. When you note the slight ideomotor movement, feel confident that you are ready for state-dependent learning. You can also use a pendulum to determine if you are in hypnosis. If you hold it between your thumb and finger and imagine it going in a circle, you will quickly learn to make it do so without any muscular movements of the wrist, hand, or fingers via the ideomotor neuron response to imagery when in a light hypnotic state.

> Ideomotor movements account for non-conscious motions of the hand-held pendulum...the intention or thought is transmitted to the motor cortex at a subconscious level, coordinated by the cerebellum, and sent down spinal nerves to the appropriate muscles, inducing micromovements not visible to the naked eye but amplified by the hand held pendulum or by the slow ratchet-like cumulative movements of a finger or other body part.[1]

Once this subtle change in consciousness occurs, begin giving yourself a single suggestion. The suggestion should have been previously determined, and it is best to learn one objective at a time. The suggestion may be in the form of a sentence or two, or it may be a visualized image of the desired result. The specific goals for self-hypnosis preparation for personal medical emergencies may vary from person to person, depending on individual needs. One person may be especially negative when reacting to the sight of their own blood. Another may lose control with the slightest feeling of pain. Still, another may have problems when the emotion of guilt or anger is involved. Generally, however, everyone should program a reaction to a serious predicament that will allow for confident and automatic access to the following:

1 An immediate, objective appraisal of the situation and injuries (i.e., primary and secondary surveys)
2 A hopeful realization that the worst is over and that you have the capability of positively coping with the circumstances
3 The belief that you can and will give yourself hypnotic directives to control applicable involuntary nervous system functions so as to increase your chances for survival

A Survival Mindset

Besides the specific objectives listed above, preparation for saving oneself during personal emergencies can include the development of a survival mindset. This is the mindset of those occasional victims at the scene of an emergency who seem to be in control no matter how badly they are hurt and regardless of the psychological intervention of the rescuer. Such a mindset is valuable not only to survive personal injury or illness but to persist when confronted with danger of any sort.

The following list gives six of the most important mindset beliefs for optimal perseverance and personal growth in the face of danger. Look at each one, and see how your current belief compares to it. If they differ, imagine (or remember) the loss of control your belief could have (or had) in a specific survival situation. Do this until the inappropriateness of such a belief becomes obvious. Next, replace this view of reality with the one that is listed. Now, using selfhypnosis, visualize the gain in control that comes from the new assumption.

With this kind of mental practice, the new belief system will automatically help you maintain control the next time fear or circumstance calls for such action.

1 *When the emotion of fear comes forth, it is better to focus on the present task at hand than on either the past or the future.* "The point of power is in the present." If you believe this, you have an inexhaustible realm of ability at your command. When thoughts are focused on an immediate task, rather than on past events or imagined futures, you become unconsciously aware of many facets of your environment. If your thoughts are in the past or future, all you will have in the present is your fear. When fear comes, let it do no more than stimulate the adrenalin for your actions. Concentrate not on the fear, but on the immediate skills, work, and action. New, positive emotions will then follow the nature of your concentration, and your fear will disappear.
2 *Everything has a humorous side, and it is always worth looking for.* One of the positive emotions that can emerge when you concentrate in the present is

laughter. A sense of humor has brought more people through difficult times than perhaps any other mental perspective. A humorous angle is embedded in all of life's predicaments. Being able to take yourself seriously and laugh at yourself at the same time is, at first, an elusive skill. But, with practice, a sense of humor will emerge spontaneously.

3 *Imagination is more powerful than determination.* Although you could walk along a 4-inch plank lying on the ground, you probably could not do this if it were suspended a hundred feet in the air, even if you were offered a great deal of money. Regardless of the knowledge that you have the ability and the determination to earn money, your imagined possibility of falling would probably be the controlling factor. Survival is seldom a matter of willpower, but of imagination to know what we ought to turn our wills toward.

4 *There are usually more than two alternatives.* There is a common mindset in which an individual automatically assumes that there are only two ways a situation can be resolved, and they limit themself to two ways of responding to a problem. This differs from the mindset that understands there are usually several ways of reacting to a particular situation.

5 *Differentiation is as important as generalization.* Generalization is a learning strategy necessary for survival. But if your belief system does not also allow for differentiation, then optimal adaptation to stress is not likely to occur. Consider the following example.

Let us say you are lost and injured in a remote area. The land is hot and dry, and there have been wildland fire danger warnings posted. You smell smoke, and, using generalization alone, you now believe, on top of all your other troubles, you are going to be caught in a forest fire. So you run in the opposite direction, becoming further lost. If your mind-set included differentiation, however, you would have considered the possibility that the smoke was from a large campfire, built by people who could have helped you. You would have looked for clues to determine the truth about the fire, and as a result, your life would have been saved.

6 *How we label things influences our reaction to them.* Labeling things is an important aspect of human communication, but during emergencies it can get us into trouble. When we label, we evaluate and predict, often erroneously. Most people are not aware of how much arbitrary labeling of situations— whether in the form of self-statements or with statements to others—can influence outcomes. With this new belief in mind, you can change problems into challenges, liabilities into assets, difficulties into opportunities, and a canteen that is half empty into one that is half full.

Exercise

Using a piece of dental floss with a paper clip tied to the end, or a pre-made necklace that can serve as a swinging pendulum, practice getting in moving via self-hypnosis and the visualization of it moving in a circle. When you get it going, you are in light trance. If you have a positive affirmation ready to go, and double-task by keeping the pendulum going while you imagine becoming confident or whatever the affirmation is, you are doing self-hypnosis. If the pendulum stops, start over.

Note

1   Shenefelt, P. (January, 2011). Ideomotor signaling: From divining spiritual messages to discerning subconscious answers during hypnosis and hypnoanalysis, a historical perspective. *American Journal of Clinical Hypnosis*, 53(3), 157–167.

19 The Planetary Emergency

The phenomenon of hypnosis may have played and may continue to play a role in our human-caused planetary crises, from climate change to pandemics. If so, it may also offer a significant solution. This chapter offers a brief argument supporting the influence of spontaneous hypnosis in behaviors causing destruction to life systems, and suggests ways to reduce or mitigate the thinking or images behind the behaviors. One of these ways goes as far as to suggest that our deep beliefs might even directly affect life systems, negatively or positively, in the same way a first-responder's words can affect the medical emergency victim positively or negatively.

Four Arrows has written extensively on worldviews. His focus has been on the non-binary, contrasting continuum that can be described as a movement between "dominant" and "Indigenous" worldview precepts. Take a moment to look at the worldview chart at the end of this chapter so as to better understand the continuum. Perhaps view the left side of the chart as our left-brain hemisphere, and the right side as our right-brain hemisphere. He believes we are out of balance with an over-emphasis on the left-side precepts.

He also believes that the human mind requires both cognitive learning and trance-based learning to maintain optimal survival. This is why, he contends, meditative mindfulness practices and continual engagement in particular ceremonies is emphasized in traditional Indigenous cultures. Trance-based healing was also a highly effective general practice, along with plant-based medicines. If maintaining an uninvestigated dominant, Western-based, post-colonial worldview is contributing to ecological destruction as opposed to the Nature-based worldview that guided humanity for most of its history, then looking at both spontaneous hypnosis from hegemonic and/or propagandistic sources would be worthwhile. Furthermore, if re-balancing calls for a stronger emphasis on the right side of the chart or the right brain (recognizing the oversimplification of hemisphere laterality that is popular), then utilization of self-hypnosis for transformations that can heal our planet would make sense.

Of course, the concept that propaganda and hegemony have a hypnotic effect is arguable. Yet quotes like those below reflect the idea that mass media,

DOI: 10.4324/9781003430261-22

propaganda, and other forms of hypnotic communication can influence people's thoughts, emotions, and behaviors in profound ways, especially during traumatic events.

Although we think that we think, most of the time we are being thought by the collective mind, the hypnosis of conditioning.

Deepak Chopra

As far as the mass of the people go, the extraordinary swings of opinion which occur nowadays, the emotions which can be turned on and off like a tap, are the result of newspaper and radio hypnosis.

George Orwell

All people who have been describing, who have been studying, mass formation, such as Gustave Le Bon, for instance William McDougall, Elias Canetti have remarked that mass formation is not similar to hypnosis but that mass formation is exactly equal to hypnosis. Mass formation is a sort of hypnosis.

Mattias Desmet

In any case, whether mass formation or group think or worldview relate to hypnosis phenomenon or not, many of the same strategies of communication for patients presented in this book can also make a difference in reversing thinking and behaviors responsible for some of the destructive insults from which our planet is suffering. Sam Keen says this more poetically in his book, *The Passionate Life*, when he says, "The terrible and promising conclusion we must draw is that we will create a world that gives us evidence to support the metaphors by which we live." In other words, we may be suffering an imagination crisis that fails to recognize the worldview assumptions we enact. Just as negative images can negate survival mechanisms in the emergency patient, negative images can also create a self-fulfilling prophecy for the planet. Similarly, as positive images can create optimal survival conditions for the mind-body complex, they may be able to influence the health and energy systems of the planet.

The new physics reveals that there are gaps and jumps in the energy continuum that defy our ordinary perception of space and time. They connect actions, places, ideas, and moments in ways that no one has been able to explain adequately. What if image-producing communication can not only influence our destructive or constructive behaviors, but can also directly affect the health of the planet? Well, first of all, we must also note that the new physics says that consciousness is a form of energy. It too, then, is interrelated to all actions, places, ideas, and moments. Since by consciousness, we are linked to everything, we also influence everything. Just as the atoms that comprise our cells are interrelated to the atoms that comprise all other structures, our thoughts are also interactive. The British physicist, Sir James Jeans, described it well as far back as in the 1940s:

> Today there is a wide measurement of agreement … that the stream of knowledge is heading toward a nonmechanical reality; the universe begins to look more like a great thought than like a great machine. Mind no longer appears as an accidental intruder into the realm of matter; we are beginning to suspect that we ought rather to hail it as the creator and governor of the realm of matter.[1]

Another way to understand the effect of our thoughts and images on the universe in and around us is to recall how a negative mood can affect people with whom you come in contact. Similarly, remember how a good mood can have a positive effect. Note that your words and body language triggered the reactions. With meditative self-hypnosis, through our thoughts, images, and daily communication, we may be able to alter the course of events that shapes the world picture.

Unfortunately, most of us have been expressing our communication in negative ways, using words that negatively influence both ourselves and all life around us. How easy this is to do when so many horrible things are being communicated to us through the media. It is important to know the truth, but when we respond, we can remember the power of the spoken word during times of stress. We can reframe the problem and change the images that are being projected.

Situation: You have just returned from a hectic commute in traffic. When you arrive home, you read on the news that the number of automobiles in your area will double in two years. Then you hear on a podcast that pollution from auto exhausts is most responsible for the depletion of the ozone layer. At this point, you will probably make a negative comment about the future of the planet. In this situation, you are the rescuer.

Man, we're not going to be able to breathe the air outside our door in five years!

With this statement you are contributing to the self-fulfilling prophesy that many others are probably duplicating at the same moment. If, however, you reframe the problem as a challenge or an opportunity with a hopeful conclusion, as you have learned to do with your emergency patients, your contribution to the mass-energy or consciousness can be positive:

You know, the pollution from automobiles has been getting worse each year. We really need to do something to make the situation better. I read about an inventor who is trying to develop the capability to economically use helium as a fuel for cars so that the exhaust would be pure oxygen. Wouldn't it be neat if the air got better because of automobile exhaust instead of worse? We'll find an alternative, don't worry.

If the writing above, based on the facts regarding imagery, positive transference, quantum mechanics, the energy of consciousness, and the impact of language, has any merit at all, then this simple reframing, if done by enough people, might significantly create an environment in which new solutions to the pollution problem will be more likely.

In addition to rephrasing the bad news into an opportunity for positive change, there are other things that you can do to help assure that your images for the planet are optimal. Of course, there are also many actions you can take. For example, recycling, buying electric cars, conserving water, boycotting companies that are irresponsible, writing your congressman when appropriate, and so on—all are important. The positive images that you hold, however, when joined with those of others, may make the biggest difference in the long run.

Guidelines for Positive Outcomes Exercise

Try your best to follow the guidelines and directives below. Perhaps you are being joined by others who are reading this book. See what happens.

1 *Surround yourself with optimistic people.* Just as living cells have structure, react to stimuli, and organize according to their own classification, so do thoughts. Thoughts thrive on association. They magnetically attract others like themselves and repel those considered to be enemies. If you spend your time listening to the criticisms, complaints, and doomsday projections of people, soon you will be joining them in this kind of communication. Ask your friends to change the subject if they cannot say something positive, or leave the room until they do.
2 *Search for a positive focus when you read or listen to radio or TV.* It may not be easy to find, but you will be surprised at how often you might have missed it in the past. More importantly, investigate the origins of your negative beliefs. Remember that beliefs are the foundation of images. If your beliefs are based on old bias or propaganda, your images will tend to perpetuate the negative effect of these ideas. This may require redefining hope so it is not about positive outcome expectations, but rather about knowing that whatever the outcome, you are doing the right thing.
3 *Pay attention to your self-talk.* You communicate hundreds of words to yourself, without selectivity, every few minutes. Some of these words reinforce negative emotions and beliefs about yourself and the world. Listen to yourself and change the negative self-statements to positive ones.
4 *Utilize the power of repetition.* It is no secret why most of us use the same words to complete the sentence, "Things go better with ----------" You do not need a multimillion dollar budget, however, to repeat optimistic statements to yourself or others often enough for them to take hold of your imagination.

5 *Take time when you visualize to do something for the planet.* Most of us use such opportunities to manage our stress, enhance our performance, or prepare for a crisis. We tend to leave the fate of the planet out of our positive images. Once in a while, take a few minutes and use self-hypnosis-type mental processes to create a positive image for the world. Be general, or use your knowledge to focus on specific solutions. In addition to the above, making a habit of the following basic qualities will promote the kinds of positive images that bring forth success. Embracing these qualities as you address the world picture will help assure that you are significantly contributing to the health of the planet.

6 *Practice optimism.* See the glass as half full instead of half empty. Turn problems into opportunities. Focus on the rewards of success rather than on the penalties of failure. Encourage and praise more often than you criticize. Help others realize that life on this planet is really worth saving.

7 *Laugh and sing more often.* Remember that laughter universal. It connects people in an obvious way. It is also contagious. Laugh daily, even if you do not think there is anything to laugh about. Neither your body nor the people around you will know the difference, and all will benefit. Also, laughing is a catharsis. So when bad news strikes, it is a good way to rid yourself of it.

8 *Be aware.* Do not avoid bad news by hiding from it. Become educated about the alternatives for positive change so you can focus your images and communication. Remain open-minded. Trust your intuition as you do your logic. Experience nature and risk adventure so that you truly feel a part of the universe.

9 *Emphasize loving actions.* Treat all living creatures with kindness. Do not exploit others. Give your time and your energy to others, and remember to start with your inner circle of family and friends. Love yourself also, and love every moment as though it were your last.

10 *Remember to think in the present progressive tense.* By "becoming" in the now you remain in control. We have no control over the past or the future, only, to some measure, of the present. Although you can have images of a positive future, and you can review pleasant memories of the past, your mental concentration is the most effective when images are "becoming alive now."

11 *Cooperate with your fellows as best you can.* A sense of commitment to the planet is important if it is to survive. When survival and growth is no longer an issue, it is a temptation to focus on our own pursuit for pleasure. Our society must remember that it was cooperation that got it to the top. Develop mutual support systems when and wherever you can.

12 *Be positively motivated rather than negatively motivated.* Focus on the rewards of a healthy planet. Concentrate on solutions, not problems. If you fear an outcome, you subconsciously set that out come up as a goal, and you

will automatically strive toward it. Remember that we are motivated by our dominant thoughts. Since either fear or desire is behind most motivation, let desire be your green light for moving forward. Fear can be used to motivate people to stop doing something harmful to the planet, but only desire will provide the alternative.

13 *Do not give up.* Be persistent. Do not be disappointed if your positive attitude does not seem to change the world. All worthwhile efforts take time (perhaps a lifetime) and persistence.

14 *Be responsible.* We are individually responsible for how we respond to events and information. There is no benefit in just blaming others. If you think a corporation is doing something damaging to the environment, take some positive action. Each of us is accountable to life. We must decide on what values we attach to it, plan on ways to uphold those values, and set goals that actualize those values. Even if your goals are never fully realized, your continual pursuit of them makes you a role model for others to follow until the goal is ultimately accomplished.

15 Have confidence in the part you play in the scheme of things. Tap your dormant resources of power and use the tools of communication to stimulate that power in others. With that confidence and your sincere concern for all others, including the planet, positive things will happen. Whether you use thoughts and words to save an emergency patient, to treat a chronic disease, to inspire a child, or to reshape the planet, it is your choice to make.

16 Study and utilize the worldview chart below using trance-based learning for appropriate transformations. Remember not to look at it as a rigid binary, but rather as a non-binary duality of apparent opposites that are necessarily a continuum with which one must seek complementarity between the precepts on the left and right and between each of the 40 precepts on both sides.[2]

Dominant and Indigenous Worldview Manifestations[3]

Common Dominant Worldview Manifestations	Common Indigenous Worldview Manifestations
1 Rigid hierarchy	Non-hierarchical
2 Fear-based thoughts and behaviors	Courage and fearless trust in the universe
3 Living without strong social purpose	Socially purposeful life
4 Focus on self and personal gain	Emphasis on community welfare
5 Rigid and discriminatory gender stereotypes	Respect for various gender roles and fluidity
6 Materialistic	Non-materialistic
7 Earth as an unloving "it"	Earth and all systems as living and loving
8 More head than heart	Emphasis on heart over head
9 Competition to feel superior	Competition to develop positive potential

(*Continued*)

(*Continued*)

Dominant and Indigenous Worldview Manifestations[3]

Common Dominant Worldview Manifestations	Common Indigenous Worldview Manifestations
10 Lacking empathy	Empathetic
11 Anthropocentric	Animistic and bio-centric
12 Words used to deceive self or others	Words as sacred, truthfulness as essential
13 Truth claims as absolute	Truth seen as multifaceted, accepting mysterious
14 Rigid boundaries and fragmented systems	Flexible boundaries and interconnected systems
15 Unfamiliarity with alternative consciousness	Regular use of alternative consciousness
16 Disbelief in spiritual energies	Recognition of spiritual energies
17 Disregard for holistic interconnectedness	Emphasis on holistic interconnectedness
18 Minimal contact with others	High interpersonal engagement, touching
19 Emphasis on theory and rhetoric	Inseparability of knowledge and action
20 Acceptance of authoritarianism	Resistance to authoritarianism
21 Time as linear	Time as cyclical
22 Dualistic thinking	Seeking complementary duality
23 Acceptance of injustice	Intolerance of injustice
24 Emphasis on rights	Emphasis on responsibility
25 Aggression as highest expression of courage	Generosity as highest expression of courage
26 Ceremony as rote formality	Ceremony as life-sustaining
27 Learning as didactic	Learning as experiential and collaborative
28 Trance as dangerous or stemming from evil	Trance-based learning as helpful and natural
29 Human nature as corrupt or evil	Human nature as good but malleable
30 Humor used infrequently for coping	Humor as essential tool for coping
31 Conflict resolution with revenge, punishment	Conflict resolution as return to community
32 Learning is fragmented and theoretical	Learning is holistic and place based
33 Minimal emphasis on personal vitality	Personal vitality is essential
34 Social laws of society are primary	Laws of Nature are primary
35 Self-knowledge not highest priority	Holistic Self-knowledge is most important
36 Autonomy sought in behalf of self	Autonomy sought to better serve others
37 Nature as dangerous or utilitarian only	Nature as benevolent and relational
38 Other-than-human beings are not sentient	All life forms are sentient
39 Low respect for women	High respect for women
40 Ignorance of importance of diversity	Aware of vital importance of diversity

Notes

1 https://www.azquotes.com/quote/721820
2 See Four Arrows's work on the CAT-FAWN Connection, where CAT stands for Concentration-Activated Transformation (Self-Hypnosis) and FAWN relates to moving from dominant ways of viewing fear, authority, words and nature to those that reflect the kinship worldview (See *Restoring the Kinship Worldview* (2022) by Four Arrows and Darcia Narvaez, selected by U.C. Berkeley's Science Center for the Greater Good as 1 of 15 books of 2022 that is "thought-provoking, inspirational and practical."
3 The chart was first published in 2020, Four Arrows book The Red Road: Linking Diversity and Inclusion Initiatives to Indigenous Worldview. The chart and extended description can be found at https://kindredmedia.org/2022/12/discovering-using-kindreds-worldview-chart-by-four-arrows-a-video-with-four-arrows-and-darcia-narvaez/

Index

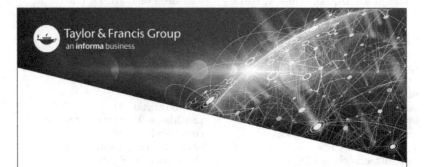

Printed in the United States
by Baker & Taylor Publisher Services